For the Benefit of Those Who See

# For the Benefit of Those of Those Who See

*Dispatches from the World of the Blind*

# Rosemary Mahoney

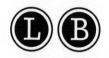

LITTLE, BROWN AND COMPANY

*New York  Boston  London*

Little, Brown and Company
Hachette Book Group
237 Park Avenue, New York, NY 10017
littlebrown.com

First Edition: January 2014

Little, Brown and Company is a division of Hachette Book Group, Inc. The Little, Brown name and logo are trademarks of Hachette Book Group, Inc.

The publisher is not responsible for websites (or their content) that are not owned by the publisher.

The Hachette Speakers Bureau provides a wide range of authors for speaking events. To find out more, go to hachettespeakersbureau.com or call (866) 376-6591.

Library of Congress Cataloging-in-Publication Data
Mahoney, Rosemary.
 For the benefit of those who see : dispatches from the world of the blind / Rosemary Mahoney. — First edition.
    pages cm
 Includes bibliographical references and index.
 ISBN 978-0-316-04342-7
 1. Teachers of the blind. 2. Blind, Workers for the. 3. Blind — Education — India. 4. Blind — Services for — India. 5. Mahoney, Rosemary. I. Title.
 HV1626.M24 2014
 371.91'109515 — dc23
                                                                                    2013025870

10 9 8 7 6 5 4 3 2 1

RRD-C

Printed in the United States of America

*For Stephen Anthony Mahoney*

To get back to the crutches, the truth about them is that they worry the onlooker more than the user.
— Flannery O'Connor, *The Habit of Being:*
*Letters of Flannery O'Connor*

# Contents

For the Benefit of Those Who See

# Vision

Not long ago I accompanied my boyfriend to Jerusalem for his laser eye surgery appointment. From Cyprus, where Aias lives, Israel is a forty-minute flight; you've hardly taken off from Larnaca's tiny airport before you're skidding to a landing again at Ben Gurion Airport in Tel Aviv. The surgery took place in the private clinic of an Israeli ophthalmologist of considerable reputation. This ophthalmologist doesn't smile much, but his mouth is slightly lopsided in a way that makes him look perpetually on the verge of a smile. He looks as though he is privately enjoying a mildly amusing joke, although after spending twenty minutes in his company one suspects there really is no joke, it's just the way his mouth is. He is short and stocky and neckless, and though his eyes are small and set close together, and though he doesn't truly smile, there is warmth in his face. He walks slumped a bit to the right, as if he has too much ballast in his starboard pocket, and moves through his clinic in a dogged way, like a weary commuter trudging through Grand Central Station at rush hour. His pending smile notwithstanding, I got the distinct sense that the surgeon was thoroughly bored with his job. At any one time there were approximately fifteen patients sitting in his waiting room, waiting for a first consultation or waiting for their surgeries or waiting, eyes bandaged, for their follow-up appointments. Each time I found myself in this room (I found myself there on three separate occasions), I could not refrain from counting the number of patients and doing a little mathematical calculation. If Aias was paying four thousand euros for his surgery, then the others probably were too. 15 x €4,000 = quite a lot. The ophthalmologist was possibly bored but certainly rich.

In first consultation, the surgeon explains the process with sentences he has used hundreds—perhaps thousands—of times before. His style is sleepily deadpan, which somehow lends him an air of incontrovertible authority. Probably because he is required to, he offers a brief overview of the possible negative outcomes of the procedure, that one-in-a-million chance that you will emerge from his surgery worse off than when you went in, that wholly far-fetched possibility that you might come out of his surgery not just your same old presbyopic self but plumb blind—or, if not blind, then at least optically diminished in one way or another.

After detailing these disturbing possibilities, the surgeon looks at you and blinks dryly, waiting for your horrified reaction. The dry blinking is a prompting of sorts, a cue, a wry indication that you have nothing to worry about, that it is extremely unlikely that you will go blind under his expert care. And so, somewhat intimidated by the entire enterprise, swept along by the rush of medical language and quite in the dark as to what it all means, a bit too polite to turn back now, the patient does not react in horror but simply nods and smiles with false detachment to show that, yes, of course, it would be ridiculous and perhaps a bit hysterical of him to think that he might come out of this costly surgery worse off than when he went in.

Before beginning his work on Aias that day, the surgeon asked me if I would like to observe the procedure from a small room adjoining the operating theater. From there, I would be able to see the surgery not only through a plate-glass window but also, highly magnified, on a television screen above the window—an exact broadcast of what the surgeon himself saw through his double-barreled microscope. Generally eager to observe just about anything new, greedy for any unusual experience, easily seduced by the wonders of modern technology, and lulled by the surgeon's dispassionate manner, I said without thinking, "Yes."

Of course, the moment I saw Aias's eye—that most vulnerable of organs—tremblingly huge on the screen, I felt that perhaps I had made a mistake in choosing to observe. Magnified a thousand times, the eyelids looked like desert dunes, the lashes like wind-tossed palms, the creases in the skin like a hundred parched arroyos. The rims of the enormous lids were raw and pink, damp and very tender-looking, the blue iris so immense it looked astral, like an exploding star, and the crimson blood vessels were dense and tangled as tree roots. How horribly exposed that eye appeared, how creepily suprahuman. In a sympathetic reaction of discomfort, my own eyes began to blink and water.

Presently a sort of screen slid across the eyeball, like a paper-thin sheet of ice, and then it crumpled and the eye was bathed in a foam of crystalline bubbles that slowly dissolved. Next, a metal clamp appeared, dug deep beneath the edges of the upper and lower lids, and pried them wide apart. And then a spade-shaped scalpel blade moved into view, hovering half an inch above the glittering eyeball. At the sight of this razor so close to the eye, I felt my face clench into a grimace, and my right hand leaped involuntarily to my throat in a nonsensical gesture of self-defense. I had made a mistake in choosing to watch, but having agreed to do it, I could not look away now—it was a matter of both stubborn pride and obsessive curiosity. The tip of the scalpel pierced the cornea at the edge of the iris and began to carve its way around the brilliant blue circumference.

I am not a squeamish person, but at the sight of this piercing it was all I could do to keep myself from shrieking and running out of the room. (The cornea, the transparent film that protects the iris and the pupil, is by the way one of the most sensitive tissues of the human body, packed with so many hotly vibrating nerves that the slightest intrusion produces an explosion of excruciating pain. If you haven't gleaned this fact from your own life's experience, you are an unusual person indeed.) With a small hook, the surgeon lifted the clear circular flap of cornea that he had, but for a small connective strand of tissue, cut free from the eyeball, and flipped it up, like the nearly severed lid of a tin can. The black pupil at the center of all this activity continued to stare straight ahead, spookily, not moving a fraction of an inch left or right, as if mesmerized by visions of an apocalyptic future.

I looked away from the screen and through the window into the operating room. The surgeon's back was to me. Dressed in a sky-blue robe and puffy blue shower cap, he was hunched over his microscope, his two small eyes pressed to its eyepieces, while a big-hipped nurse stood slightly behind him in the posture of a lobster—elbows crooked and lifted slightly away from her body, gloved hands raised near her ears, and a swab of cotton pincered between the thumb and forefinger of each hand. Several inches beneath the bottom lens of the microscope, Aias's face was bathed in a pool of intense orange light. The surgeon's gloved hands basked and darted in the pool like fish in a tank. More disturbing things happened in this surgery: drops of liquid were flung rudely into the eye, cotton swabs were raked across the eyeball, an intensely bright and vibrating laser strobe light circled around and around the dilated pupil, and all of this in a manner that seemed blunt and savage. It was like watching a seal pup being torn to shreds by a ravening shark.

At some point I realized that in my distress, my left hand had joined my right hand at my throat to assist in the self-defense, as if perhaps I was expecting the scalpel to jump out of the screen and take a stab at *me*. I watched the surgery but tried not to perceive it, saw the violated eye but tried not to comprehend it, yet it was impossible to remain calm while viewing this lurid physical anathema.

The surgical hook appeared again and fitted the slick layer of cornea back over the iris with a jaunty little flip of dismissal: *Ho-hum, that one's done. Next, please.*

I stared, fixated. What would keep the almost severed cornea in place now? What would prevent it from falling out and dangling on Aias's eyelash when he stood up?

From the corner of my eye I saw a rapid blur of motion near the window. It was the surgeon; he had turned toward me and was waving his scalpel in friendly greeting. Having caught my attention, he gave me a wink above his surgical mask and added to it a jocular little hula-esque swing of his hips and the double thumbs-up sign to show that all had gone well with the first eye.

The surgeon, though he didn't smile, was kind of a humorous guy—an actor of sorts—and maybe, I thought, a touch peculiar precisely because he did not smile as he made these vaudevillian gestures. Though his mouth was hidden by the mask, it was obvious from the steady, lightless look in his eyes that he wasn't smiling. His nurse, however, was smiling liberally behind her mask—her eyes narrowing a fraction and transmitting a sudden excited illumination the moment her boss began doing his little dance.

The surgeon must have seen that my face, as I'd been looking up at the screen, was twisted into a grimace. He must have thought I was nervous and afraid and must have been trying to reassure me. If that was what he was thinking, he was quite right: I was nervous and afraid, because I, for one, have a morbid fear of losing my eyesight.

*     *     *

When I was a senior in college I was playing squash with my friend Vicki one cold February evening when she wound up powerfully for a swing and, in the process, struck me square in the right eye with her racquet. The blow was so sudden and unexpected that I had had no time at all to close the eye, and the edge of the racquet scraped roughly across my exposed eyeball. I felt a hot pain that seemed to razor into my eye, go through my brain, bounce off the back of my skull, and ricochet back and forth that way several times. I covered the eye with both hands and dropped to a crouch, knees to my chin, for perhaps half a minute, during which Vicki's hand fell on my shoulder and rested there sympathetically until, after getting no response from me, it sheepishly withdrew. She said my name a few times and asked if I was okay. I was unable to answer. As my silence and her worry mounted, she began to apologize in a voice of rising alarm, and her hand fell again to my shoulder, this time patting profusely. Finally I straightened up and tried to open the eye. It was impossible. The pain was too great, and when I opened it for a fraction of a second I saw nothing at all but the sharp white light of the squash court. "Shit," I said. "Shit."

Holding my elbow, Vicki guided me out of the court and walked me through the snow to the student health clinic several blocks away. In our hurry to get help, we had left our street clothes in the locker room and were out in shorts and sneakers. It had begun to snow. I remember the hissing sound of the evening traffic on the wet pavement and the feel of the snow landing against our bare legs in an effervescence of icy prickles. The pain in my eye was not like any pain I had felt before. It was as if a hundred grains of broken glass had been ground into the eyeball. I walked with my head bowed and one hand cupped over the eye. I knew that Vicki felt guilty and sorry, and to try to make her feel better and to hide my fear, I made some joke about going blind, but the joke was feeble because I knew from the volume of pain I was experiencing that whatever had happened to my eye was quite serious and that perhaps it really had been permanently blinded. That thought crept into my consciousness, and now I was beginning to have a hollow feeling of irrevocability, of the impossibility of reversing time and fate. One minute my eye was healthy and keenly following the trajectory of a squash ball, the next it was not and I was stumbling down Massachusetts Avenue with my hand clapped protectively over it.

At the student health clinic, a doctor thumbed my eye open in a way that seemed unnecessarily brusque while a nurse flashed a bright light into it. The doctor said, "You will have to see a specialist." It wasn't the gravity in his voice but the quickness with which he said it that frightened me. The nurse gave me a painkiller, put a gauze pad over my eye, then guided me outside to a waiting taxi and told the driver to take me to the Eye and Ear Infirmary at Massachusetts General Hospital. Vicki insisted on coming with me; I insisted that she not. I didn't tell her that having company with me on a medical errand always felt like a burden heaped upon another burden. Under duress, I didn't want to have to focus on my companion, to worry about her mood or whether she was becoming impatient or to feel guilty for taking up her time. I have always preferred to suffer alone.

I sat in the back of the taxi with my hand held lightly over the bandage. The familiar streets sliding hazily by before my good eye looked only half familiar, and in my heart I knew that I would spend the rest of my life this way, seeing everything in monovision, missing half my visual perception and therefore half the world.

This happened thirty years ago but I still remember the doctor's last name: Cobb. Dr. Somebody Cobb. He was youthful and fit and by coincidence he knew my mother, had examined her eyes just a few months before, a fact that I found inordinately comforting. I remember that he put an anesthetic in my eye to numb it, dilated both my pupils with eye drops that streamed down my cheeks, pressed my face into a thing like a stereoscope, shone bright little lights into my eyes, and, finally, pronounced the cornea deeply torn. It would take several weeks for it to heal itself. He taped a patch over my eye and released me.

Because both my pupils had been dilated, when I left Cobb's office, everything was a mushy blur. Even my healthy unpatched eye was useless. A nurse accompanied me through the revolving front door of the hospital, wherein I caught my sneaker between the moving door and the jamb, lurched forward, and banged my forehead smartly on the glass, an indignity that under any other circumstances would not have made me cry but that under these circumstances—insult added to injury—brought hot tears of frustration to my helpless eyes. The nurse said, *There, there, now,* with a not unkindly hint of riddance and handed me over to a taxi driver, who guided me by the elbow from the spinning door of the hospital, through the jumbled darkness, and into the backseat of the car. The cold seat shocked my bare legs as I slid myself onto it. As the driver drove me back to my apartment in Inman Square, the lights of the city smeared past the wet car window. Once home, I stumbled my way immediately to bed.

I remember the depth of the gloom I felt as I lay there that night. It wasn't the unfathomable pain I experienced every time I moved my eye right or left or up or down but the certainty that my eye would never be right again. It made no difference that the doctor had said the cornea would heal. I didn't believe him. How ignominious to be blinded by a squash racquet. How ignominious to be blinded by anything at all. What horrible luck. It gave me a dank, sinking feeling of dread. I imagined being totally blind forever and how unbearable that would be and began to panic a little.* To be blind would be to become one of those people I had always pitied and slightly feared, one of those people who through no fault of their own had been deprived of their vision and, thus, their real enjoyment of life, their effectuality, their potential. That it was no fault of their own somehow made the tragedy worse.

Most of us who have healthy eyesight are extremely attached to our vision, often without being conscious that we are. We depend heavily on our eyes and yet we rarely give them a second thought. I, at least, am this way. The physical world is almost hypervivid to me. The appearance of objects is registered instantly and boldly in my mind with no conscious effort on my part. I cannot help noticing tiny details. I have a friend—and not a stupid one—who once spent an entire lunch with a man and never noticed until the very end of it when she moved to shake his hand that he was missing his right arm. How, I have several times asked her with real bafflement, was that possible? Such a thing could simply never happen to me. Ever. I would have noticed within fifteen seconds if that man was missing merely a button on a shirt cuff. I would have noticed whether he had hair in the spaces between his knuckles, would have noticed the length of his fingernails and exactly what shape the fingernails were. I would have noticed the

---

*No, not just a little—a *lot*. A few years before this event I had seen for the first time the film version of *All Quiet on the Western Front*. One scene had stayed vividly in my mind: In the midst of a relentless bombardment, a band of German soldiers are putting up barbed wire to keep the enemy at bay. The younger ones are wild-eyed with fear. The bombardment worsens, and the soldiers are directed to retreat to their dugout. As they go, one of them gets knocked to the ground by an explosion and the next thing we know he is screaming hysterically, "My eyes! My eyes! I can't see! I'm blind!," and running around in jagged circles. The very next thing we know, he's dead. It isn't entirely clear what has killed him, but I think we're meant to suppose it's the injuries he sustained. I knew better, though. I knew in my heart that the soldier had died not of his injuries but of the sheer horror at knowing he'd been blinded. I had felt his utter despair, his psychic repulsion, so forcefully that I frowned at the television screen and said out loud, "It's *better* that he died."

color of his eyebrows, the size of his ears, the condition of his teeth, the quality of his hair and skin, and all of this without making a conscious effort to do so. If one person in a group of ten is missing the tip of his little finger, I will notice it almost immediately.

This extreme attention to visual detail is not a virtue, just a fact of my person. It happens seemingly involuntarily and strikes me as neither good nor bad. Possibly (because I don't seem to be able to control it) it's a neurosis. Or maybe it's just evidence that I am at heart a shallow person who can't help fixating on inconsequential surface details. Certainly it's superfluous. It doesn't help me at all, I don't need it to survive, and yet my eyes are always searching for information. I will spot an acquaintance on the street, a friend in the supermarket, an old classmate on a subway long before he or she has spotted me. I always remember a face. If I meet a person once, I will remember the face four years later, remember where I first met the face, what other faces were present, and what was the mood of the meeting. I will likely not recall the name, but the face I will remember.

But seeing and noticing aren't a function of the eyes alone. They are as much a function of the mind, and in my case, perhaps they aren't as involuntary or superfluous as I tend to think. On further consideration, I suspect that my mind could not really operate without my eyes, because in fact it is my mind that is constantly asking questions of the visual world, looking for evidence, for information, judging existence on the basis of what I see. In me, it's a kind of tireless vigilance and possibly even a defense. I am like a security camera ever on the watch. The furtive quality of vision feels to me like an incredibly valuable weapon. Everything I see gets transformed into a private sketch or painting in my mind, stored away for future reference, future evidence, future ammunition. I fear that my mind would starve and that I might find myself in danger if I had no visual information, that it's chiefly the light, the shapes, the spaces, the colors that I see that compel me to keep moving forward in life and that keep me safe. The first time I read John Berger's *Ways of Seeing*, I was struck by the sentence *We only see what we look at.* I believe that what Berger meant by this was *We see only what we look at.* But the sentence seems to me as significant in its other interpretation: We, alone, know what we are looking at. Unless some keen witness is watching every movement and focus of your eyes, you alone know what you choose to see and perceive. The employment of vision is private and even covert. And, of course, the beholder chooses not only what he will look at but what he will make of what he sees.

Lying in my bed that terrible night thirty years ago, I concluded that being blind was worse than being dead. Being blind was like lying alive within a locked coffin. I'd be trapped and hidden in that dark box but able to hear the world outside carrying on entirely without me. Blind, I'd be left behind. I would want to hammer on the lid of the coffin and shout, *For Christ's sake, let me out!* but my arms would be pinned to my chest in that tight space and all I'd be able to do was scream. But the screaming would get me nowhere. I'd be imprisoned that way for the rest of my pointless life, conscious of my predicament and helpless to change it.*

Surely being blind was like being buried alive. I was certain then that I would rather die than lose my eyesight.

Aias came out of the surgery with hard transparent plastic protective covers taped over his eyes and moving a bit unsteadily at the side of the surgeon. I hooked his arm through mine and led him across the waiting room, in which that day there sat a preponderance of Hasidic

---

*Years later, when I read in Leonardo da Vinci's *Paragone* that a man who had lost his sight was like "a man shut alive inside a tomb where he could live and move," I thought that if he had only removed the second clause, his description would have been dead accurate.

women. Some wore heavy loaflike wigs that gave them an armored appearance, and those wigged women who had bandages on their eyes looked particularly baleful. As we moved toward the door, the surgeon gave me a startling nudge in the ribs with his elbow. "What about you?" he said. "You want the surgery?"

I laughed with false agreeability and nodded in a way that meant *Oh, sure! Good idea! Thanks for thinking of me* while in my heart I was thinking, *Fat fucking chance. You wouldn't catch me dead submitting my eyes to that knife.*

For a while Aias had been encouraging me to have the surgery. He hated it when I reached for my eyeglasses, hated the way they looked on me. But even though it was true that at age forty-nine, I found my eyes rapidly weakening, I was adamantly set against laser eye surgery. I couldn't read a thing now without magnifying lenses, not unless I squinted severely and held the text as far away from my face as my arms would allow. I often heard myself muttering with ornate irritation, "I cannot see a *thing* anymore." And yet I would rather be dependent on eyeglasses and the annoyances of losing them, sitting on them, endlessly wiping fingerprints from them, replacing the loose screws on them, rummaging constantly in my bag for them or thrashing my way through the house in search of them when in fact they are sitting atop my head the whole time, silently mocking me—I would rather endure all those minor annoyances than surrender my eyes to anybody or anything over which I could not have complete control.

The surgeon said his unsmiling good-byes and admonished Aias not to exert himself unduly for the next forty-eight hours. We took a taxi back to our hotel, where Aias lay on the bed, head propped up on three pillows, hands by his sides, nose and toes pointing at the ceiling. With the bulbous protective cups over his eyes, he looked somehow incarcerated, detained. In an hour or so I was to remove the coverings and put medicinal drops in his eyes. It struck me as I looked at him lying there that being sightless was akin to being toothless. Self-defense and aggression both seemed to me difficult to achieve fully when you had no eyes or teeth. For a few seconds I imagined Aias toothless, his mouth caved in. Which would I prefer him to be: toothless or blind? Toothless looked bad, but then some kinds of blindness did too. Toothless was a condition that could be remedied with a bit of expert dentistry, whereas in most cases blindness could not be remedied by anything at all.* I sincerely hoped that Aias was not blind. Soon enough, when I administered the eyedrops, we would have the answer.

I went to the window and looked out. I could see Jerusalem's old cemetery on the hill to the north. The stones of the tombs gave off a parched, senile yellow light and looked, from this distance, for all the world like the rubble of a ruin. A phalanx of stiff-spined cypress trees stood at the edge of the cemetery as cars crept by on the avenue below it—Israelis going about their business while the skeletons above them lay motionless in their tombs, a silent reminder of what was ahead for all of us.

Bored, I lay down on the bed next to Aias and held his hand. I knew he disliked being idle and debilitated. But he was a patient person, far more patient than I. Had I been in his position I would have been restlessly bad-tempered, complaining bitterly, and emitting dark vocal sighs of despair every sixty seconds or so. Aias, however, was silent and relaxed, waiting for time to take its course. He could even smile at his predicament, showing his strong teeth. I smoothed his knuckles and fingers, put my arm over his chest, kissed his neck and ear. I admired

---

*Later, I'll discuss some of the cases in which sight has been surgically restored to the congenitally blind. The earliest reported instance came from Arabia in the year 1020. By the year 2000, there had still been only a very few successful cases.

his patience and his equanimity. He made it easy to take care of him. I pressed my cheek to his, kissed him on the mouth. He kissed me back. The call to prayer suddenly began quavering from ten different directions outside our window, and we lay that way for a long while until one thing led to another and even though the surgeon had said that Aias should not exert himself in any way, we exerted ourselves. Gingerly we did so, and while we did, I was very careful to keep my hands away from his face, fearing I would damage his eyes.

Eventually, Aias's eyedrops were due. I settled my eyeglasses on my nose and carefully peeled away the adhesive tape that held the protective plastic covers in place. The eyes were filmy and watery. Aias blinked and looked beyond my head in a testing way, trying to focus. I held his eyelids apart and put three drops into each eye. The liquid pooled, then streamed from the corners of his eyes and slid toward his ears. When his eyes cleared he looked at me for a while, minutely examining my face. Finally he said what I knew he would say: "Those glasses you're wearing are no good."

Surprised and relieved that he could see me through all that rheum, I said, "How come?"

"They make you look old. They make you look like an old schoolteacher."

Just around that time I had, in fact, become a schoolteacher of sorts. I had recently taken a job as a volunteer teacher at the International Institute for Social Entrepreneurs in the city of Trivandrum in the state of Kerala in southern India—nearly as far south in India as a person can go without stumbling off the end of Cape Comorin and plunging into the Laccadive Sea. The school was not exactly in Trivandrum but eleven miles outside the city in what seemed to me a deeply insignificant coconut and banana jungle set between a tiny village and a muddy lotus-choked lake called Vellayani. Housed in a walled brick compound of brand-new construction, the school comprised four buildings—an office building, a dormitory, a dining room/kitchen that also served as an auditorium, and a classroom building. I was there to teach English and anything related to it. Communication, pronunciation, elocution, writing of all forms, grammar, punctuation, public speaking, whatever the students needed in this broad area, I was to help them with it. Not having had more than two years of experience with this sort of thing, and that nearly twenty years ago, I was only one step ahead of my students. There were some two dozen students between the ages of twenty and fifty-two. They came from thirteen different countries. There were two from Madagascar, three from Kenya, one from Norway, two from Ghana, one from Japan, one from Colombia, one from Nepal, three from Germany, three from Liberia, one from Sierra Leone, one who got chased out of Liberia as a boy and ended up in Sierra Leone, one ethnically Indonesian man from Saudi Arabia, two technically Chinese people from the Autonomous Region of Tibet, and one irrepressibly cheerful, fast-talking young woman from so extremely far northeast in India she might as well have been Bhutanese.

One of the criteria for admission to this school was that the student be proficient in English. For a couple of the students, that criterion appeared to have been waived. Though they could all put together simple sentences, only a few were truly proficient in English. The Kenyans' national language was English and they were, of course, fluent in it, though their English was full of quirks and Britishisms and their accents were so rich that one had to concentrate carefully to follow what they were saying. The Liberians, for whom English was also the national language, were also very good at it. They knew English, understood it perfectly, but when they spoke it, they were almost completely unintelligible to the rest of us English speakers. No amount of careful concentration could solve this problem. The number of times

I had to say "Sorry, what did you say?" to my Liberian students in the first few weeks of meeting them was a source of regret for me. I felt for them. With their nation, their lives, their education, their very psyches disrupted and dismantled by Charles Taylor's nightmarishly weird Liberian civil war, they were not like any of the other students at the school, and they felt their difference and were, I eventually came to realize, quietly wounded by it.

The other important criterion for attendance at this school was that the student had to be either legally or entirely blind. Thirteen of them were completely blind. The rest were in various stages of blindness, low vision, or visual impairment. Some could see a little light, a little color; some could see objects dimly; a few could read printed type if the type was very large and they pressed their noses up to the page. Most could read Braille; most were in possession of a white cane.

My reason for going to India to teach blind and visually impaired people was not that I wanted to teach English or live in India. I have never really wanted to teach, and I might as well say now that, although I've tried over the years to see the charm of India, after five separate trips there—a couple of them extended—I still do not see the charm of India. No, I was teaching at this school solely because I had developed a strong curiosity about blindness and wanted to meet blind people, to spend time with them, to get to know them, to find out how they think, to see how they live in the world, how they navigate, how they talk and eat and dress and write and shave and brush their teeth, and learn just about anything else I could about blind people without trespassing too far beyond the limits of decency. Teaching in a school for the blind seemed to me a good way to learn, and I was given the rare chance to do that in Trivandrum, Kerala.

I had begun to develop this interest in the blind four years before, when an American magazine sent me to Tibet to write an article about Sabriye Tenberken, the blind German woman who, together with her sighted Dutch partner, Paul Kronenberg, founded Braille Without Borders, Tibet's first school for the blind. At the time that I went to Tibet, I had no real interest in blindness beyond the usual reflexive dread of it, the usual pity for people who couldn't see, the usual fearful wish that it would never ever happen to me. My dread of blindness was great enough that I was even a little apprehensive about meeting Sabriye. In preparation for my trip to Tibet I read a book she wrote about her experiences and saw photos of her (she looked normal enough, presentable enough; when I accidentally held her photo upside down for a moment, she looked oddly like me when I was younger); she was by all accounts a brave, adventurous, highly intelligent person, but still, she was blind, and that big, terrible fact made me uneasy and even reluctant to meet her. I didn't know what was the appropriate way to behave with a blind person, whether there was some particular etiquette I should follow. There must, I thought, be rules about relating to a person so extremely disadvantaged in the game of life. The unfamiliarity of it worried me and the bleakness of it depressed me a little. I was forty-five years old at the time and had rarely spoken to a blind person.

My first encounter with a blind person took place thirty years ago in the waiting room of Raidió Teilifís Éireann, the Irish broadcasting company in Dublin. I was sitting on a couch waiting to do a radio interview when a blind woman came into the room with a guide dog and sat down next to me. She was moonfaced and pale and wore a red dress and black patent-leather shoes. Her thin hair was cut in blunt bangs across her forehead, and over her ears she wore the bulky headphones of a Walkman that she held lightly in her right hand. The guide dog lay on his side and stared dully at the woman's glistening shoes while she listened to music with her eyes closed. Her eyes were slightly sunken, and the lids had a darkish hue, as if lightly dusted with coal ash. I was enthralled by the pair. The woman's nose twitched repeatedly, as though she were investigating a breeze or a scent that was wafting across her face. Presently, a short bald man poked his head through a doorway and said to the blind woman, "I suppose you'd better come and operate the switch, Lisa." She unplugged the headphones from the device, removed them from her ears, stuffed them into her handbag, then abruptly lifted the Walkman to within an inch of my chin and, with bold authority, said, "Pardon me, madam. I want to be sure the machine is off. Is it off?"

Startled, I took the machine in my hands, fumbled with it, accidentally turned it on, turned it off again, confirmed that it was off, and handed it back to her. She said, "Right, then," and stood up and headed for the door with no guidance from the dog, who followed slowly behind her with an air of resigned obedience.

I remember wondering with intense puzzlement how the blind woman knew that I had been sitting there, for I had not moved or spoken or made any sound at all since she came in and sat down next to me. And how was she going to operate the RTÉ switchboard if she didn't know whether her own radio was on or off? Above all, how did she know I was a woman? She had called me madam. Why? With strong feelings of suspicion, mistrust, fascination, and resentment I watched her and the dog disappear through the doorway.

Aside from one fleeting exchange with a blind man over the harness of his guide dog in a very small elevator in Boston, a vacuous little volley of small talk in which neither the blindness nor the conspicuous dog was mentioned, Lisa had been my only real encounter with a blind person before I went to Tibet. Fourteen years later, on my way to Lhasa I felt that my ignorance about blind people could somehow hurt both them and me.

Affixed to the great door was a beautifully handwritten note that said BE AWARE OF THE DOG!, which is a euphemistic way of saying THERE IS A VICIOUS DOG IN HERE WHO WILL PROBABLY BITE YOU. More often than not, though, it's really only a way of saying THERE IS NO VICIOUS DOG IN HERE, BUT WE WANT YOU TO THINK THAT THERE IS. Whatever the case, merely being aware of a dog is of no use at all if the dog is determined to attack. I hesitated, considered the possibilities, heard nothing beyond the door but the raucous clatter and shriek of children at play. Realizing that after traveling some eight thousand miles to write an article about this school, I didn't have much choice, I rang the bell, an ancient-looking bronze cowbell dangling from a rope. I waited, staring at the magnificent gate. Had a winged, fire-snorting Chinese dragon come roaring out of it, I would not have been entirely surprised. Eventually the great doors were hauled open by a tall, skinny teenager in a double-breasted pin-striped suit jacket three sizes too big for him. He was smiling hugely, positively brimming with delight. One of his eyes was rolled back in his head and the other seemed to be looking intently westward. The sleeves of his jacket dangled several inches below his hands, making him look like an amputee.

The school's courtyard, a little smaller than a tennis court, was full of blind Tibetan children of varying ages and sizes. Some were kicking a ball around; some were singing along with a Dolly Parton tune on a cassette player parked on an outdoor staircase; one boy, stripped to the waist, was washing his hair at a spigot in the corner of the yard; several were wrestling on the ground; one plump girl was descending a long flight of outdoor stairs with a pile of laundry hugged tight in her arms. Two boys were sitting in the sunlight at the bottom of the front stoop, snapping sheets of bubble wrap held close to their ears. A girl in a pink jacket with its hood pulled up over her head stumbled out through a doorway, leading by the hand a smaller girl in sky-blue sneakers.

The scene had the cheery abandon and unself-conscious intimacy of a Brueghel village panoptic. Some of the children had damaged eyes; one or two had no eyes at all; some had eyes that didn't open. Others seemed to be able to see a little bit of light with one eye or the other. One boy of about six with a Band-Aid on his forehead was standing in the middle of the yard with his face lifted to the sky, his thumb and forefinger curled into a circle around his left eye, like a monocle, and his mouth twisted into a grimace of extreme effort as he struggled to catch a glimpse of the enormous sun. Many of the children had white canes. A serious-faced, big-eared boy of about thirteen with an orange down jacket, orange trousers, and a head shaven nearly to baldness sat in the sun on a wooden bench worrying a set of Tibetan prayer beads, eyes closed, lips moving. He wore black leather brogues with thick heels and big square metal buckles on their tops, the sort of shoes in which the persecuted British pilgrims clunked about on the decks of the *Mayflower* in 1620. With the shaven head, the orange clothing, and the beads, the boy resembled a Buddhist priest. He seemed unaware that at the end of his bench a large Tibetan mastiff with an enormous head lay locked in a wire cage. The Tibetan mastiff is a famously aggressive dog so frighteningly tough and hardy that he can happily sleep through the night buried under a few feet of snow.

Distracted by the sight of the children, I didn't realize at first that the blind teenager who had opened the gate was standing expectantly beside me, still grinning, waiting for me to identify myself. His double-breasted jacket seemed part of a costume, like the jacket of a dandified 1940s gangster. I thanked the boy for letting me in and said I was here to see Sabriye Tenberken.

At the sound of my voice, the entire yard of children immediately stopped what they were doing and turned their heads in my direction. Silence replaced the school-yard din. It was obvious from the way the children's expressions suddenly changed, from the way they stood statue-still and tilted their heads at me, that they knew I was someone new and knew exactly where I was standing in relation to them. After a long silence, I said, for want of anything better to say, "Hi, kids," whereupon several of the children began to approach me slowly, their faces keen with curiosity, their chapped cheeks not just pink but raw-beef red, as if rasped by the powerful sun. Their hair was raven black and glossy as shellac in the intense light. They surrounded me and began to run their small hands over the hem and sleeves of my coat, the legs of my jeans, and my hands. I said hello to them, and hearing English, they began to question me in English. They told me how nice it was to meet me, wanted to know my name, where I was from, why I was here, how I was feeling today. At the sound of our conversation, the rest of the children gathered around and they, too, began to feel my clothing. Their warm hands were all over me, gently exploring with a soft tap-tapping, like airport security guards frisking for weapons. They felt my shoes, my ring, my fingers, my belt, my legs, my handbag, their hands doing for them what their eyes could not. The children were open and bold and yet shyly respectful at the same time. I was a newcomer, but they seemed to have no real wariness of me—instead, they approached me as if I were a novel object. Those who could see a little light squinted a lot as they talked to me. One boy gave me his full name with a regal nod of his head. Another boy with no front teeth and eyes crazily skewed in their sockets held my hand and said, "I am six years old." He looked no more than three. Later, as I came to know the children better, I understood that they were all small for their ages.

The only child in the yard who didn't come to investigate me was the boy on the wooden bench, the monk with the prayer beads. Through it all, he continued to pray, lips moving, eyes closed, fingers stitching at the beads, an expression of serious inertia on his long face. He could not have cared less that a stranger had arrived. Either that or he was deaf as well as blind.

The six-year-old who was missing his front teeth shook my hand with determination, then felt the watch on my wrist. He held my wrist to his chest, and, with fingertips that moved pickingly, like the feet of a spider, he thoroughly examined the watch and its strap. His breath was hot and moist on my knuckles. He lifted his red cheeks at me. "Watch, is it?"

"Yes," I said. "It is."

He pressed the watch to his ear, and, holding his breath, he listened awhile, his mouth hanging open in concentration, his unseeing eyes, a bit too big for their sockets, rolling a little in his head. Again he showed me his cheeks. "Time?"

"Eleven o'clock."

"Morning eleven, is it?" he asked fervidly, if a bit disingenuously, for he must have known it was morning.

"Yes."

"O'clock?"

The questions, I realized, were just an opportunity to practice his English vocabulary. "Of course o'clock," I said, "what else could it be?"

Summarily dropping my wrist, the boy said, "Tchah! Time to go in."

As the children began to file back into their classrooms, Sabriye Tenberken came out of the main office building with a white cane in her hand. I introduced myself to her. Her eyes were striking. They were stark blue, clear, deep-set, and, although they saw nothing at all, they were vibrant and healthy-looking. When I spoke, she faced me directly and gazed with such focused concentration she seemed to be not just seeing me but seeing through me. She didn't *look* like a person who couldn't see. She was tall and slender, had an angular, Roman sort of beauty: a high forehead, a long nose that came to a marked point, blond eyebrows, dirty-blond hair, and pale flawless skin. She was dressed in jeans and a red fleece jacket. She spoke fluent English with a German rhythm but very little accent. After asking politely whether I had settled into my hotel (I had), whether I found it com-

25

fortable (I did), and whether I was tired after my long trip (I was), she told me that she was just on her way to run an errand and invited me to join her on her walk to the center of the city. She talked a lot and with energy and confidence, and I understood immediately that she is a person who is always busy, that she rarely idles.

The second thing that struck me about Sabriye was her style of walking. She has notably long legs and walks quickly and with a kind of urgent authority. Indeed, she strides, which was not the gait I expected from a blind person. Apparently accustomed to walking arm-in-arm with companions, she hooked an elbow in mine and, linked in this way, I found that for every step she took I had to take a step and a half. Quickly I understood that on this particular occasion she had linked arms with me not in order for me to guide her, but so that she could guide me.

I had been in Lhasa less than twenty-four hours, and the city's high altitude — nearly twelve thousand feet above sea level — and consequent reduced atmospheric pressure had made me breathless, light-headed, and physically clumsy. Not forty seconds into our walk, I stumbled over a pile of granite stones that had been dumped in the middle of the sidewalk. Sabriye, who just at that moment was saying, "People always ask me when did I go blind, " interrupted herself to steady me, then carefully guided me to the edge of Chingdol Dong Lu, a central four-lane artery on which heavy traffic with an extreme form of disorder unique to China (and India) careered by in both directions.

Sabriye lifted her chin a fraction, cocked her head in concentration, waited for a break in the two lanes of eastward-rushing traffic, then led me swiftly to the dead center of the avenue, where, to my dismay, we paused atop the yellow dividing line. Large trucks roared past so close to us that the wind they whipped up tossed Sabriye's long blond hair across her mouth as she spoke. "But I can never say when exactly I went blind," she said, the white cane held lightly in her fingers, her voice rising to compete with the noise of the traffic. "It was gradual. I began to realize that a color I thought was green was really blue. I couldn't see words I was writing. I thought I could see, but I couldn't."

A small break appeared in the two lanes of traffic rushing west, and at just the right moment, Sabriye applied a light pressure to my arm and we plunged forward and crossed safely to the far side of the street. There, without breaking stride, she hopped nimbly over a knee-high barrier that separated the bicycle lane from the rest of the traffic and stepped up onto the sidewalk. She turned left at the next corner, where a woman selling steamed dumplings from a bamboo pot stared at her in astonishment. I could hardly blame the woman, for I too was staring, mystified as to how Sabriye managed to navigate the world so swiftly and flawlessly. She hurried across a vacant lot in which six pool tables had been set up under the vivid blue Tibetan sky, turned slightly left again, went straight for a minute, veered around a pile of rubble, somehow dodged the bicycles blowing past us in the narrow alleys, turned left again, then right. Because our elbows were still linked, I had to maintain a hectic little skipping trot to keep up with her.

As we barreled up yet another narrow street, a wiry little fox-faced girl sitting on a stoop spotted Sabriye through the crowd, sprang to her feet, and crowed at the top of her lungs, *"Xia ze lai le!"* A simple Chinese sentence that means, in essence, *Here comes an idiot!*

Sabriye repeated the words to herself with a dry laugh and carried on. "Nobody can insult me with blindness," she said lightly, "because I'm proud to be blind."

Almost single-handed Sabriye Tenberken and her partner, Paul Kronenberg, brought literacy to the blind people of Tibet. In founding Braille Without Borders, they inspired nothing short of a revolution in the status of the Tibetan blind, in their thinking, and in their future. She and Kronenberg, who is sighted and handles much of the practical work of the school, were knighted by the Dutch queen and won numerous other honors and awards for their work. Sabriye was hardly an idiot. Nevertheless, in the seven years she spent living in Tibet— and, indeed, in the twenty-seven in her native Germany before that— she had been the object of abuse, epithets, and condescension innumerable times because of her blindness. These days, epithets left her unfazed; they hadn't always.

Sabriye was born with retinitis pigmentosa, a degenerative disease of the retina, and by the age of twelve, she was completely blind. In her early years, she was able to make out faces, colors, even landscapes, but her vision was highly impaired, and as a result her schoolteachers approached her with what she felt was a patronizing deference that set her apart. They always shook her hand first in the morning when the students arrived at school, always offered her the biggest piece of cake at lunchtime. They spoke down to her and singled her out for special treatment because she was blind. Her classmates, by contrast, taunted and ostracized her, played tricks on her, bullied her and deliberately gave her misinformation and false directions in order to watch her tumble down a flight of stairs. They told her she was ugly. Unable to see her own face, she believed the lie. Desperate to fit in, Sabriye denied her blindness even to herself and worked overtime to hide it. At bus stops, she would ask bystanders to read the bus schedules for her with the excuse that she had something stuck in her eye. Or she simply got on the wrong bus, too proud to ask where the bus was going. Out of sheer determination she continued to ride her bicycle long after it was reasonably safe to do so; more than once she and the bike ended up in a ditch. Observing how clumsily she moved, people would ask her if she was drunk. Once, skating on a frozen lake, she skated out of the prescribed safety bounds and fell into a hole in the ice. Sabriye averred that not accepting her blindness made her miserable, for she was constantly compensating and pretending, exhausting herself in the effort. Eventually she met a girl whose vision was approximately as diminished as her own. The girl told Sabriye that she walked with a white cane. When Sabriye said, "A cane is for a blind person," the girl, who had fully accepted her own blindness, responded, "But I *am* blind."

"Not until I accepted my blindness," Sabriye told me with visible emotion, "did I begin to live."

Sabriye's parents enrolled her at the Carl-Strehl-Schule in Marburg, a boarding school for the blind where, along with the usual academic subjects, the students were taught horseback riding, swimming, whitewater rafting, Braille, and, above all, self-reliance. Suddenly, Sabriye realized that as a blind person she was not alone, that there were many others like her. She made friends. She felt equal and appreciated. She was happy. She learned Braille and for the first time in her life, she read an entire book by herself. She read *Dr. Faustus* and the works of Shakespeare. She thought, *Okay. I may be ugly and blind, but I have a brain. I can do things.* It was at this special school for the blind that Sabriye began to learn that her blindness need not be an obstacle, that it need not set her apart from sighted people or cut her off from the world or prevent her from having a happy, fulfilled life. She developed a newfound confidence. At sixteen, at a party, she was invited to dance by a boy who didn't know she was blind. Before long, the boy asked her if she was having trouble seeing. When Sabriye answered, "I'm blind," the boy told her that her blindness made him uncomfortable and he stopped dancing with her. Sabriye said to him, "If you have a problem with my blindness, you don't deserve me."

Eventually, Sabriye attended the University of Bonn, the only blind person in a student body of thirty thousand. She majored in Central Asian studies with a particular focus on Tibet. Several professors in the department tried to dissuade her from studying the difficult Tibetan language. No one had yet found a way to translate Tibetan into Braille and therefore there were no Tibetan texts available for the blind. How, then, would she read the assignments? How would she keep up in her classes? How would she make notes on the required Tibetan texts? Sabriye ignored their discouragement and immersed herself in her courses. Using the system of rhythmic spelling that Tibetans employ to memorize their complex language, she created her own method of translating the Tibetan language into Braille. With a specially adapted Braille writing machine, she found she was able to take notes faster than her sighted classmates. She compiled a Tibetan-German dictionary, and when sighted students began asking her for help with their course work, she was vindicated and delighted. Eventually, Sabriye helped to devise a software system that enabled her to transcribe entire Tibetan texts into formally printed Braille.

Sabriye had developed the system for her own use but when she realized that blind people in Tibet could benefit from it, she got the idea to bring it to Tibet and start a school. In a pattern of skepticism that even now Sabriye faces daily, almost all of her professors told her that her idea was absurd, that although what she had accomplished so far was remarkable, it would be completely impossible for a blind woman to take on such a project. They told her to be realistic, to keep her feet on the ground; they told her not to give false hope to the blind, not to imagine that she, a blind woman, could accomplish something so revolutionary and grand in scope.

Sabriye ignored the objections. She approached several development organizations for help with founding her school in Tibet, but all of them saw her blindness as too great a liability. After having numerous doors closed in her face, she resolved to realize the project under her own aegis. In 1997, at the age of twenty-six, much to the dismay of everyone but her immediate family, she traveled alone to China, took an intensive course in Chinese, then proceeded to Tibet, where she was surprised to learn that more than thirty thousand of Tibet's 2.6 million people were blind—about twice the global rate. While poor diet and unhygienic conditions contribute to the high rate of blindness in Tibet, the main cause is the country's elevation. At such high altitudes, the sun's ultraviolet rays are intense and cause damage to the unprotected eye.

Sabriye also discovered in Tibet a deep prejudice against the blind. Tibetan culture is rife with superstition, mythologies, ghosts, vapors, and spirits. Blindness is rarely considered the result of anything so banal as genetics, disease, or neurological disorders. Most Tibetans believe blindness is caused by mysterious powers or spiritual forces as punishment for misdeeds perpetrated in a past life. The blind are considered to be cursed, possessed by demons, or capable of extrasensory perception, which makes them entirely dangerous; in parts of Tibet, it's thought that merely touching the blind can cause a person to become impure. For centuries Tibet's blind have been shunned, vilified, treated as subhuman, and subjected to unimaginable cruelty. When Sabriye first arrived in Lhasa, she found not a single institution or organization geared toward providing assistance for the region's blind—clearly a result of this deep-seated fear and enmity.

Sabriye decided to travel through remote areas of the Tibetan countryside, visiting rural villages, spreading the word about her Braille system, assessing the situation of blind children there. Many of these villages were not accessible by road, and when Sabriye concluded that the most efficient way to conduct her mission was on horseback, there were more howls of protest from the skeptics. Nevertheless, she set off with three supportive companions, two of whom were Tibetan, and rode from village to village, across high mountain passes, and through flooded rivers. What she found in her investigation shocked her: a small child who, because of her blindness, was tethered to a bed most days, her tiny body withered with misuse; others, barred from the local schools, who regularly had stones thrown at them, who were taunted and jeered at and locked in dark rooms for years on end. Isolated, scorned, sometimes beaten and abandoned or turned out in the streets to beg, almost all were uneducated and completely illiterate.

When villagers saw Sabriye walking and confidently riding a horse and heard her speaking Tibetan, they refused at first to believe that she was blind. With patience and persistence she persuaded them that she was indeed blind and that their blind children also could learn to ride horses, could learn to read and write and speak foreign languages. Gradually comprehending the truth of what Sabriye was saying, one astounded Tibetan father told her, "The prospect of your school is like a dream for us."

With twenty thousand dollars of Sabriye's own money and with fierce determination, Sabriye Tenberken and Paul Kronenberg finally managed to set up a school in a rented building in Lhasa. They began with six students. Six years and a host of trials later, the school now had thirty-seven students in residence, ranging in age from three to nineteen, as well as six trained teachers and five staff members. New students arrived regularly.* The school charged no tuition or boarding fees; it was a free ride for whatever motivated blind student could present himself at the door. Paul and Sabriye paid the bills by applying for grants and traveling a great deal to make speeches and raise funds from private sources. Against all the odds, Braille Without Borders was a success.

While Sabriye and I walked, the sky had begun to fill with bloated plum-colored clouds. Explosive thunder cracked around us. The

---

* By 2013, 250 students had benefited from the Braille Without Borders program.

Tibetan sky is so close to the ground that the thunder seemed to roll just a few feet above our heads. The noise was huge and crisp and so violent it sounded like a four-poster bed crashing willy-nilly down a long flight of wooden stairs. It rattled the windows of the shops and drowned out our voices. Sabriye shuddered, visibly disturbed by the sound, and for the first time she hesitated in her path.

"I can't stand loud noise," she said.

Surprised, I said, "It's just thunder."

"Yes, I know. It's harmless, but I find the noise overwhelming. I hate, for example, construction sites. When I hear a jackhammer, I break into a sweat of anxiety. Noise is my only real fear."* She resumed walking and said with a small, self-protective laugh, "The only other thing I'm afraid of is vampires."

I was sure I had misheard her. "Vampires?"

"Yes. I have a vampire phobia. I hate myself for it, but I have a vivid imagination. Sometimes when I'm walking at night I hear footsteps following behind me and I never care whether it's a criminal or whatever, because I studied karate and street fighting for a year and a half and I know I can defend myself. But the moment I think, *Maybe it's a vampire,* I feel a real panic."

She blamed the fear on her older brother, who as a child had had a mania for vampires. He knew every last detail about them and insisted on sharing the details at length with Sabriye. At a certain age, the brother began sleeping in a coffin. He watched countless vampire movies on television, and, because he knew that Sabriye was afraid of

---

*Fear of noise is common among the blind. The blind French author Jacques Lusseyran described the phenomenon in his memoir *And There Was Light.* "For a blind person, a violent and futile noise has the same effect as the beam of a searchlight too close to the eyes of someone who can see. It hurts." By the way, Lusseyran's memoir of his involvement with the French Resistance contains a description of life in a German concentration camp that is more vivid and affecting than any other account I have read.

them, he would force her to watch the movies too. "He loved to go to cemeteries, and sometimes he would bring me with him," she said. "For him it was a thrill; for me it was absolutely terrible. I loved my brother, but those vampires really scared me."

I wasn't sure how to respond to this. I wanted to tell her that her vampire phobia was absurd and that her brother sounded like a complete creep. But she was blind, and I was a visitor at her school, and so instead, I said politely, boringly, "Well, I can understand your fear. But do you still think vampires exist?"

After a long silence she said with a smile, "No, I don't really think they exist. But, you know, Tibetans believe very much in ghosts and spirits. You can easily draw yourself into thinking like that here. I can sometimes believe in ghosts in Tibet."

Another explosive thunderclap boxed our ears and made us jump. I realized that I was completely lost now in the heart of the city and that I would not have been able to find my way back to the school without Sabriye's guidance. As we proceeded through the narrow streets, I continued to be amazed by Sabriye's navigational skills, by how completely assured she was in the back alleys of Lhasa. In the span of forty-five minutes she never once collided with anything or took a wrong turn. Her hands never groped or darted, either investigatively or defensively. She never hesitated or stumbled. She walked in a smooth, gliding way and seemed always to know at what moment to turn left or right. It was like watching an elaborate trick performed by a particularly talented magician. Mystified and amused, I finally asked her how she did it, how she knew where to turn, how she knew she had reached a corner without touching the wall, how she knew when there was a person or a parked truck in her path.

"Well," she said, "lots of things. Sound, echo, the air, different smells—these things change around you and you know from experience what they are."

From the way she spoke, it was obvious she'd been asked this count-less times before and that for her the answer to my question was so elementary that having to give it yet again was a bit tiresome. She told me she could hear how wide a street was by listening to the echo of her cane tapping on the pavement, how wide a staircase was by clapping her hands or snapping her fingers as she ascended it. "You know," she said, "sighted friends of mine who knew me well told me I should not come to Tibet to try to take this project on, because when they shut their eyes and see darkness, they feel completely helpless. They couldn't imagine how I would do it. But for a sighted person who closes her eyes and suddenly tries to live life that way, it's not the same experience as for a blind person who has had years to adapt and learn and com-pensate. Sighted people don't understand that. They don't understand what the world is like for a person who has long been blind."

Sabriye went on to observe that most human beings are attracted by beauty, that we make quick judgments about people based on their appearances, but that for blind people this sort of superficial judgment simply isn't an issue. "A blind person's reason isn't clouded by appear-ances. We have to focus on the personality, which is the real essence of the person. It can be an advantage for us."

In order to illustrate this point Sabriye sometimes asked sighted vis-itors to the school to join her for tea in a completely dark, windowless room in the school basement. "We leave the lights off and introduce them to other new people there in the dark. We have tea and conver-sation, and the sighted people have to make their judgments of these new acquaintances based on what they hear rather than on what they see—it's all voice, ideas, personality. Then, when we take them outside and they can finally see the people they've been sitting with, they're sur-prised, because the people look nothing like what they had imagined."

"It's not unlike making an assessment of a person just from hearing them on the radio," I said.

"Right. The radio can be a very intimate and immediate way of knowing a person."*

I had been watching Sabriye's face as we walked, reading it for clues. There is in her expression a constant mood of expectation and wry amusement. She smiles easily and speaks with casual directness. She is genial, focused, passionate about her cause, and uses a great deal of visual description. She will tell you that a person blushed, a landscape was beautiful, a lake was turquoise, a film she "saw" was frightening. There's a refreshing lack of performance in her persona, no overweening eagerness to please, no calculation, false intimacy, or apparent guile. She looks directly at you when you speak and listens with an air of such intelligence and alertness that you find yourself regretting you're not a more articulate, more vibrant person.

When we returned to the school and were passing through the small courtyard, Sabriye stopped at the mastiff's cage, reached in, ruffled his ears, and greeted him with a few affectionate words of Tibetan. The dog was lying on his side, languishing in the small cage, with his mouth open and his big tongue draped over his jagged molars. "His name is Pookie," Sabriye said proudly. "Unfortunately we have to lock him up because he's a little vicious. He bit a Swiss woman who was visiting us."

The dog struggled heavily up to a sitting position and gazed at us. He had a very large head and opaque staring eyes. I estimated that he was nearly the size of a yak. The bristling mane of hair that grew in a ruff around his neck was not unlike a lion's. His paws were as big as teacup saucers. I knew that the Tibetan mastiff was considered one of

---

*In his memoir *Touching the Rock*, John Hull, a British professor of religion who lost his sight at age forty-two, remarked on the "amazing power of the human voice to reveal the person" and maintained that he could "often hear many things which the speaker may not know are there." Similarly, Jacques Lusseyran wrote of his exceptional ability to read personality and mood in voices. "A man who speaks does not realize that he is betraying himself."

the most ferocious dogs in the world. I did not find it at all unfortunate that he was locked up.

Sabriye said, "Put your hand in the cage and pat him."

I looked at her to see if she was being funny. It was hard to tell, since she always seemed to have a slightly ironic smile on her face.

"Sabriye," I said, "do you really think I would be inclined to stick my hand into this dog's cage when you've just told me that he's a little vicious?"

She laughed. "Don't worry. He can actually be very sweet. Pat him. You'll see."

I crouched down and looked at the dog. The bars of his cage seemed dangerously flimsy. He lifted his eyes at me in a frighteningly noncommittal way. As far as I could tell, he was neither a sweet dog nor a sour one, neither happy nor annoyed to see me. He revealed nothing of his mood or temperament. Our relationship could go one of two ways. "I don't think so," I said.

Sabriye laughed again, but this time the laugh had the electrical edge of a cackle to it, an undercurrent of wicked delight. "You're afraid!" she said. She was clearly amused by my fear, which surprised and interested me. If she could laugh at someone else's expense, then surely she was fair game for the same in return. When I understood this about her, when I realized that she had just given me permission to tease and push her, I felt for the first time at ease with her. She was not the dreary, pitiable, earnest person that I had persuaded myself all blind people must be. She had, to my surprise, a sense of humor. She tapped the cage with the tip of her cane and goaded me on. "Come on. Don't be afraid," she said dismissively. "Just go ahead. He won't bite you."

"Being afraid of a vicious dog is entirely reasonable," I said. "Being afraid of imaginary creatures like vampires and ghosts is not."

Sabriye laughed loudly at that. "Okay, you're absolutely right," she said, relenting.

I put my hand reluctantly into the dog's cage—ready to retract it in an instant—and patted his big bony head. Nothing happened. The dog didn't respond, but he continued to gaze impassively at me in a way that seemed ominous. "Good dog," I said insincerely. The dog blinked once; I withdrew my hand and stood up. "Okay," I said. "I've patted your vicious dog. That's enough of that. Are you happy now?" My hand felt greasy; I wiped it on my jeans.

"You see?" Sabriye said. "He doesn't really bite."

"He doesn't *really* bite. Okay, that's good to know," I said and made a mental note to steer well clear of him in future.

The Braille Without Borders school comprised two single-story L-shaped buildings that were configured in such a way as to create this pleasant and very private little courtyard. Like most of the buildings in Lhasa, they were made of mud brick and painted white with colorful trim, and every window had at its top that narrow, pleated length of cloth. The courtyard was cloaked in mauve twilight now, and the air had grown chilly enough that I wished I had a hat. Lights had come on inside the school, transforming its many-paned windows into bright rectangles of orange. The smell of roasting yak meat drifted from the school kitchen. The courtyard was empty but for two bigger boys who were laughing as they dragged a sack of cabbages to the kitchen door.

Sabriye invited me to sit with her in her office. As we passed through the school's small dining room, I saw the boy I had come to think of as the Monk, the one dressed in orange with the buckles on his shoes. He was sitting alone at a table, still worrying his beads, his head bowed and his lips still moving in prayer. There was something extremely remote about him, as though he had no awareness whatever of his surroundings, and I began to wonder if he was not indeed blind *and* deaf.

As we headed down a hallway, I asked Sabriye about him. "Which boy?" she said moving quickly in front of me.

"The one all dressed in orange. He's sitting alone in the dining room with a set of beads."

She slowed her pace a bit and said "Oh" in a grave tone. "That's Dawa. He's very new here."

"Is he praying or just talking to himself?"

"No, he's praying. He prays constantly."

"He looks miserable."

"He *is* miserable."

When we sat down in her office, Sabriye explained that Dawa was thirteen years old and had recently lost his vision to some disease, that he was in the classic phase of depression and denial that most sighted people go through when they go blind. He refused to accept that this was his fate, which left him in a limbo of inaction and paralysis. To make matters worse, he had been told by a Tibetan fortune-teller that he might regain his sight, and although that chance was very slim, it was a hope he was desperately clinging to. He prayed constantly to effect this miraculous reversal of fate. "His uncle brought him here, thinking we could help him. He had heard that there were happy blind children here who were learning. But Dawa doesn't want to participate in anything," Sabriye said. "I've tried to talk with him about it. I told him, 'Okay, maybe the fortune-teller was right, maybe you *will* regain your sight. But for now you can't see, so you might as well do something with that. It can't hurt you to learn Braille like the other kids.' But he refuses."

I told Sabriye that I would certainly feel the same way in his situation, that I would find it impossible to get used to suddenly being blind, and that if I were in Dawa's position, I would not want to engage in anything at all. She reminded me that she too had gone through the same anger and misery and loathing, said that it was only natural, but that the boy would not really be able to start living until he accepted the fact that he was blind and began to deal with it.

"Dawa doesn't realize that there's so much he could be doing right now, because he's placing all his hope in the future and all his value in his eyes." She shook her head with concern. "It'll be hard to shake him out of his passivity."

Sabriye sat back in her desk chair and toyed with the wrist strap on the end of her cane as she spoke. She explained to me that one of the greatest obstacles for blind children, not just in Tibet but everywhere in the world, is that they are seldom treated equally with sighted children, that they are perceived as being helpless, as somehow special and different. "In families and the community beyond, very little is expected of the blind child. This reinforces in them the feeling that they are useless and incapable. Special isn't good either way. When blind kids come here, we expect something from them. We teach them Braille, Chinese, English, computers, mathematics, and navigational skills. Many who come here have been so neglected and thought so helpless that they don't know how to wash themselves. We teach them personal hygiene. We expect them to work hard at their lessons, to work hard at communal chores, to help each other out. When they first arrive they object and say, 'But I'm blind! I can't do that!,' because this is what they've been taught in their villages: *You can't. You are unworthy.* But when they realize that the other kids here are working and experimenting, being independent and gaining useful skills, they change their views. They begin to see that independence is empowering. That makes them want to work."

Sabriye told me about a blind girl named Kyila, a recent graduate of Braille Without Borders who was now training to be a masseuse and often helped out at the school. Kyila had grown up in a small village in extreme poverty. Her father was blind and so were her twin brothers. The four of them were perceived as thoroughly useless, not to mention accursed. They were bullied by the villagers and told, "You people might as well all kill yourselves because you have absolutely no future."

Kyila came to Braille Without Borders, studied hard, learned quickly, and had recently won a scholarship to study in England for a year.

"Kyila is brilliant," Sabriye said, "but nobody in her village ever paid enough attention to her to see that. Now she'll be one of the first blind Tibetans ever to leave China."

During the conversation, my notebook had been sitting in my lap. Occasionally I picked it up and jotted something down. This time, when I picked it up and began to take notes, Sabriye said with mock exasperation, "Again you're writing what I've said!"

I looked up at her, alarmed. "How do you *know* I'm writing?" I said.

"The way you lowered your head."

"How do you know I lowered my head?"

She shrugged. "I just know."

"I would only know that you lowered your head by actually *seeing* you lower it. You couldn't possibly 'just' know. You're blind."

Sabriye smiled; she seemed to be relishing the mystery.

"Well," I said, "are you blind or aren't you?" I had actually begun to wonder.

She laughed. "I really *am* blind. Completely. I cannot see you. I cannot see anything."

"So, if you're blind, how do you know that I lowered my head?"

"You were talking when you bent your head to write. I could hear the direction of your voice change in a very particular way."

"But that's a change so subtle that I would never be able to hear it in another person. And how do you know I didn't just bend my head to examine my fingernails? How do you connect it so assuredly to the act of writing?"

"I've had so many people interview me and have heard it so many times, I know what that direction means."

So, she knew what a writing voice sounded like. It was uncanny. And still I wasn't sure I believed that she was completely blind. I had noticed that wherever I stood or sat in relation to Sabriye, she always looked directly at me when she or I spoke. If I moved, her head turned to follow me. If I stood behind her, she turned a hundred and eighty degrees to look at me. I mentioned this to her, and in my voice I heard a challenge, an overtone of impatience and doubt that sounded to my own ears rude.

"This is something I've learned. Blind people who haven't been trained often speak to a wall, because they don't know how to follow the voice of the person they're talking to. It doesn't matter to them as long as they're heard. But if you want to be effective, if you want to connect to people, you can't be putting your face to a wall while you're talking to them. To a sighted person, that looks very strange. So you have to learn to read by sound where a person is in relation to you, what direction they're faced in."

"I understand," I said, and as a final personal test, I gave her the finger and held it up for quite a while, hoping to provoke the sighted person's reflexive response. She didn't react, didn't seem to notice, just continued to talk. I felt thoroughly weird sitting in this blind stranger's office boldly thrusting my middle finger at her. I dropped my hand to my lap, and when she had finished talking I said, "Let me just ask you this one thing: How many fingers am I holding up right now?"

She exhaled through her teeth in amused exasperation. "You really don't believe I'm totally blind, do you?"

"No," I said. "I do. I believe you. I'm just surprised by how extremely attuned you are to what's around you."

"The thing is," she said with a wry little smile, her brilliant blue eyes looking directly at me, "I actually do know how many fingers you're holding up."

"Really?" I said. "How many?"

"None." She laughed at this raillery and gave her desk a little slap.

"Good guess," I said.

# The Blind Leading the Blind

I sat with a group of the blind children at a long table in the dining room at Braille Without Borders, waiting for an informal beginners' Braille class to start. The room, appointed with three long wooden tables and accompanying benches, was dark and cool, lit only by the sun coming through its tall windows. Like all the rooms in the school, this one was fancifully detailed in the candy colors of a carousel—the door was a pattern of fire-engine red and royal blue, the window frames were dandelion yellow, the trim boards were sky blue, and the lower half of the walls were tangerine orange. The paint finish, even on the walls, was of a gloss so high and extreme that the colors glistened like ice. The building had once belonged to relatives of the thirteenth Dalai Lama and was obviously very old. The plaster ceiling was supported by ancient wooden beams so beautifully crooked and bowed, they looked more like a carefully designed work of art than architectural underpinnings. On one wall hung a large, full-length mirror, which seemed to me a superfluous accessory in a school for the blind. In the corner stood a box that held students' white canes.

I sat at the end of the table, near the windows. On a shelf behind me I saw a book: *The Little Mermaid,* in Braille, edited by Sabriye Tenberken and printed by Braille Without Borders. Through the window

I could see Pookie, the vicious mastiff, lying on his side in the dirt, baking in the midday sun.

Across from me at the table sat the Monk in his orange clothing. He had wrapped his prayer beads around his wrist, giving them a rest, and was sitting with both elbows on the table and his head propped up heavily in his hands. He was so removed from what was going on in the room, so seemingly oblivious, that he looked doped. His lips were moving, and for the first time I heard what he was saying: *Om mani padme hum,* over and over again in a droning monotone. He had long ears and long fine hands. Beside the Monk sat an intense, sober-faced little girl named Dolma who, according to Sabriye, was a member of the Kampa tribe. The Kampas were fierce warriors and horsemen, wild, proud, nomadic, and given to wearing elaborate headdresses and ornate jewelry. Dolma's mother had been a prostitute; her father had disappeared. One day when Dolma was three or four, the mother got fed up with having to care for her blind child and simply abandoned her by the side of a road. Eventually some Kampa horsemen happened upon the sobbing girl, and, taking pity on her, they took her in, fed her, and bought her warm clothing. Somehow the horsemen had heard about the blind school in Lhasa. They traveled a very long distance on horseback to bring Dolma here. They arrived at the school, got off their horses, dropped the girl in the courtyard, and, without ceremony or explanation, turned on their boot heels to leave. Annoyed at their presumption, Sabriye (who can be fearsome when angry) chided the men and told them how rude it was of them to just dump their child there without discussing it with her. Wounded, the horsemen wept and pleaded that Dolma was not *their* child, that they had only found her crying in a ditch one day, and that they just wanted to help her. (I pictured the proud horsemen tremulously backing away from Sabriye, wringing their hands in distress and mopping their tears with the tails of their braids.)

True to her Kampa nature, Dolma—who at that moment in the dining room was gnawing feverishly on the end of a pencil—was a bit mischievous and unruly. When she arrived at the school, she had told the other children, "I'm a witch," because her mother had insisted that this must be the case, otherwise why would she have been born blind? As a result, the other children had avoided her. The first time I saw Dolma, I thought she was a boy. There was little to differentiate the girls from the boys at this young age. They all wore the same sort of sturdy pullovers and trousers, and their black hair was cut short in a unisex style. Dolma's blind eyes had a slightly eerie aspect. They put me in mind of a pair of eyes moving furtively behind the oval holes of a Halloween mask.

At the far end of the table sat Panden Tsering and Kileh, two boys I was already acquainted with. I'd sat in a car with them on the long ride to Lhasa from Shigatse, where Sabriye and Paul had established a small farm to train blind adults in agriculture and farm management. Arriving at the farm, Sabriye and Paul and I had found these two young boys sitting all alone in the kitchen—having heard about the Braille Without Borders project, their families had simply dropped them there a few days earlier. Panden Tsering was six and Kileh was fourteen, too young to stay long-term at the farm. Sabriye invited the boys to return to Lhasa with us so that they could attend the school, and without hesitation, both boys said they would be very happy to come. We were three unfamiliar foreign adults, yet when it came time to leave Shigatse, the two boys climbed eagerly, smilingly, into the car with us. They had never been in a car before. They had probably never traveled more than forty miles beyond their homes. They carried nothing with them. No luggage, no diverting toys or gadgets, no toothbrushes; they had nothing at all but the clothes on their backs. Though they knew that Lhasa was far from their home and that they wouldn't see their families again for months, they made no protest and voiced no regret during the arduous ride over rutted roads. I marveled at their level of trust and realized I did not know a single American child who would willingly do what they were doing. During the ride I asked Panden Tsering if he was happy about going to the school; the face he made in response said, *Are you nuts? I'm thrilled!* When I asked Sabriye why these boys would join us so trustingly, she answered, "They have nothing. No friends, no future. Perhaps they're so low they feel they have nothing to lose."

Now they both sat smiling at this dining room table in the middle of Lhasa. Across from them sat a boy who had his trousers on backward. Beside him was a child with his sneakers on the wrong feet and the hems of his trousers tucked into his socks. Beside me sat the youngest child in the school, a three-year-old boy named Nimen Penzo. Fresh out of toddlerhood, Penzo had the face of an irritable grandfather, an adamant, stumping way of walking, a penchant for climbing anything within reach, and a devilish habit of striking out at people's legs as they went past him.

I had noticed that when the blind children were sitting idly together, they always sat huddled close and draped about one another—arms slung around necks, elbows linked, heads gently touching, hands entwined with hands—and I began to understand that when they held hands, they were not simply holding hands in the way that you and I might hold hands (were we to actually know and like each other) but were, more accurately, holding lightly *on to* one another's hands. This constant connecting of hands was not just a gesture of affection but a form of communication, a way of conveying and receiving subtle emotions and even ideas, much the way sighted people convey emotion or thought with glances and facial expressions. The children's eyes reflected nothing of their moods or thoughts but rolled uselessly, like milky blue marbles. It was only their hands and their voices that revealed them.

Presently the door banged open and the teacher, a boy named Kyumi, came importantly into the room. "Now," Kyumi announced in English as he crossed the floor, "we learn Tibetan alphabet!" Kyumi was twelve years old, but like many of the children here, he looked four years younger than his age. Unlike the others, he had the fussy, no-nonsense manner of an overworked forty-year-old. Kyumi was completely blind. His pants were so big they were slipping off his hips, and every thirty seconds or so he clutched impatiently at their waistband and hitched them up. He had a large head and big ears that protruded from the margins of his face like opposing handles on a sugar bowl. His wide, rosy-cheeked face was roughly the shape of a pie plate. His skin was carnation pink and pretty as a girl's. His one visible eye was glassed over with a film of unnatural glacial blue, and the other eye was rolled downward into its inner corner, which made him look as though he were trying to analyze the flare of his own nostril. Periodically Kyumi would flap his hands in the air in a rapid violent shaking fashion, as if trying to rid them of flames or caustic acid.* He had been a student at BWB for the past four years.

"Rose?" he said to me. "You are here?"

"Yes, I am."

Briefly Kyumi explained to the other students that I was an Amer-

---

*What Kyumi was doing with his hands is one of many common habits known as blindisms. Blindisms are most often displayed by blind children but sometimes by blind adults as well. They include repetitive behaviors like rocking or swaying, spinning in place, continuous rubbing or pressing of the eyes, and rapid flicking of the fingers. (Note the marked way that Ray Charles and Stevie Wonder sometimes wag their heads as they perform—this, by their own admission, is not just excitement about the music but a form of blindism.) The scientific consensus about blindism is that the lack of visual stimulation causes the energetic blind person to engage in this sort of physical self-stimulation. The gestures of blindism—like the untrained blind person's unwittingly speaking to a wall—appear to the sighted as bizarre or comical and are often interpreted as signs of either retardation or mental instability. Blindisms have no doubt contributed to the stereotype of the blind as mentally impaired.

ican girl who was not blind but wanted to learn Braille, and then, with no time to waste in further small talk, he got to work passing out pages of Braille. Kyumi moved with great purpose. He crossed to the far side of the table, put the page down, put his hand on Panden's shoulder, ran his hand down the boy's arm until he found the boy's fingers, then planted the top of the boy's index finger firmly on the Braille text in front of him. *"Ka!"* Kyumi cried, the first letter of the Tibetan alphabet.

Panden bent over the table, his nose touching the page, and he minutely examined the tiny bumps of Braille with his fingertip. *"Ka!"* he said.

Kyumi felt his way to the next boy and repeated the process. Eventually, all the heads in the room were bent low in concentration. Kyumi's teaching style was both lordly and intimate. Like all the veteran students here, he could operate a Braille typewriter, a computer, could dress and wash himself, was learning to cook, and could speak English and Chinese in addition to his native Tibetan. Though his voice was high and loud, his English had a British diplomat's precision and flourish. He spoke in a kind of shriek, wrapped his arms around students' shoulders, pressed his forehead against theirs, and entreated them as if it were a matter of national importance to repeat after him. He moved from student to student, tsking and sighing and muttering as if overburdened with responsibility, yet it was clear he relished his status as one of the quickest students in the school and was deeply pleased to have been deemed capable of passing on his superior knowledge. Everything Kyumi did, he did vehemently, precisely, and with a hint of hauteur. I had seen him earlier using a Braille typewriter in one of the classrooms. He stabbed the keys in a punishing fashion, throwing his whole upper body into the effort, and after each strike of a key, he raised his hands theatrically high away from the machine, as if fearing the keys might strike him back. I had heard him speaking Chinese;

he spoke it in a ringing voice and with an accent so perfect and grand he sounded like Generalissimo Chiang Kai-shek roundly denouncing the Communists as he fled for Taiwan.

The new students were getting the hang of the alphabet, sounding out the letters and smiling at their own fingers sliding over the pimpled pages before them. They sat with their heads bowed so low to the paper that they appeared to be listening to it. *Ka, ka, ka,* they said again and again.

Kileh began speaking excitedly to Kyumi in Tibetan. There was a brief exchange between them, and when it was over, I asked Kyumi what the boy had said. Kyumi lifted his head at me abruptly, as if he'd forgotten I was there.

"Rose?" he said, stepping toward me with his hands raised. He reached for my forearm, held it in both of his hands, put his face near mine. "That boy has said he has already studied some small Tibetan alphabet in his village."

"A little bit of the alphabet, you mean?"

"Yah, yah, yah, a little bit," Kyumi said, waving his hand at me with a dismissive flourish to indicate that it was foolish to mince words over such a trifling matter. He told me it was his pleasure to help me, then paused a moment to rest a sympathetic hand on my shoulder. "Rose?"

"Yes, Kyumi."

"Can you listen now and learn while I teach these men and women?"

I apologized for the interruption, promised it would not happen again. Kyumi wagged his head and said with a kind of noblesse oblige, "No problem, Rose. But..." And raising a correcting finger at me, he added with undisguised concern about my intellectual abilities, "Please *try* to listen and learn."

I promised him I would try, and we returned to our studies. Like the rest of the students, I shut my eyes and ran my fingers over my

page of Braille and tried to make sense of it. The feel of the sharp little dots embossed on the page was pleasing to my fingertips, but the
dots were so small and arranged in such seemingly complex ways that
I could not imagine ever being able to differentiate one dot from the
next or one letter from the next or even one line from the next. I did
not try. I drew the palm of my hand flat across the page—it felt a little
like the surface of a worn asphalt shingle. Penzo, the little boy sitting
beside me, had rested his forehead on the edge of the table and was
feeling his page with both hands, murmuring into his lap the sounds
of the Tibetan letters.

The door swung open again, and Mingmar, a thin, mischievous girl
of twelve, flew into the room chewing gum with the insouciant flair
of a swindler. The sound of communal singing coming from a nearby
classroom followed her in. She slammed the door shut and greeted her
classmates by howling at the ancient ceiling, "Friends! Nice to *meet*
you today!"

Startled, the students lifted their heads and turned in the direction
of the voice. Mingmar's elbow happened to brush mine as she passed
me, and a sudden shock of interest flashed across her face. Her hand
reached out and gently touched my knee. Like all the children here,
she had a tactile ability that was so acute she knew instantly, just from
the feel of my trousers, that I was a stranger. She stilled her gum chewing, stepped closer, put her two small hands lightly on my forearm,
and examined my cuff, my wrist, my fingers, my watch. Her eyes were
two cheerful slits; her small mouth open with curiosity. I could see the
gray lump of chewing gum perched on her tongue. After acquainting
herself with every part of my person within reach, Mingmar held her
face very close to mine and whispered softly, "Who are you?"

I told her who I was. Her face ignited with pleasure. She leaned
back on her heels and crossed her arms on her chest and said, "How
do you do, Rose! Are you blind?"

I told her that I was not blind.

With palpable pride she responded, "I am yes blind! And you are lovely."

I asked her what made her think I was lovely.

She said, "By voice I know!"

Mingmar wore a jean outfit embroidered with daisies. She had a short, harum-scarum haircut. The hair seemed to be flying every which way, vying for space on her small head. Mingmar drew herself up suddenly, and I saw that she sensed that someone was sitting across from me. She stretched her hand tentatively across the table. It collided with the Monk's elbow. At Mingmar's touch, the Monk opened one eye. Exhaustion and depression seemed to prevent him from opening the other. He did not lift his head out of his slender hands.

Mingmar turned her face to me in puzzlement. "Who," she whispered, "is this one?"

I was about to say *That's the Monk,* but I stopped myself. Before I could give his proper name, Mingmar had felt the beads on the boy's wrist, and, smiling with recognition and nodding sagely, she said, "Aha, it is Dawa." Then, leaning close to me she added very softly, "Rose, he is praying. *Om mani padme hum.*"

Mingmar listened awhile to Dawa praying, and then, quite unexpectedly, she put a foot on the bench, hoisted herself clean up onto the table, crawled across it on her hands and knees, forcibly removed Dawa's hands from his head, and pressed his fingers to the Braille paper in front of him. She said something fervid and sharp to him in Tibetan. It sounded distinctly like *Come on, you son of a gun! Quit moping and get down to work!* And then she stretched out flat on her back on the table between us, placing her head on my page of Braille. Her eyelids were nearly shut. All I could see was a whiteness as bright as typing paper in the slits between her lids. She turned her face toward me, and her small smiling mouth worked her little wad of chewing gum with sumptuous pleasure, smacking and snapping with great involvement. She crossed one knee over the other and casually bobbed her foot in the air like a woman idling on a park bench. The toe of her sneaker swung dangerously close to the Kampa girl's forehead. Mingmar let out a sigh that I can describe only as the embodiment of contentment. "Rose?" Mingmar said.

"Yes?"

"I should say that I like you very much."

"I like you too, Mingmar," I said, which was true. Mingmar was a saucy little thing and had about her a delightful atmosphere of verve, warmth, curiosity, and intrigue. I'd liked her immediately. Mingmar sealed our friendship by reaching out and patting my arm in a motherly way. Unsolicited, she began to teach me how to count to ten in Tibetan. Upon hearing my voice reciting Tibetan numbers, Kyumi instantly appeared behind the Monk, looking extremely cross. He reached over the Monk's shoulder and gave the table a loud, stern slap with the palm of his hand. Unable to see the slap coming, Mingmar and the Monk jumped in surprise.

"Rose!" Kyumi cried. "You are not learning numbers today. You are learning Tibetan alphabet. *Ka! Kha! Ga!*"

Still supine, Mingmar barked at Kyumi in Tibetan. Kyumi barked back at her. And then, perhaps to establish his seniority and thus his authority in the room, Kyumi proclaimed in English, "I am sixteen years old."

In a flash Mingmar sat up on the table, knocking the Monk's page of Braille to the floor in the process. She turned in the direction of Kyumi's voice, her little spade-shaped face slack with utter disbelief. A dark silence followed while she gathered her thoughts. Then, anchoring her hands on her hips, she cried indignantly, "No! He is not sixteen. He is only twelve. And I am too very twelve."

The beleaguered Monk slid his chair a few inches closer to the window, away from the fray. Taking advantage of the distraction, he re-planted his elbows on the table and fit his head back into his palms, this time with the fingers of one hand fitted delicately over his useless eyes. Settled back into his customary position, he emitted a sigh of complete inanition. His was not a case of mere indifference but a depression so consuming, he was unable to concentrate on anything else. The nascent hair on his close-shaven head fairly glittered in the window light.

A heated exchange ensued between Mingmar and Kyumi, during which the other children at the table turned their faces in the direction of the shouting. The irritable little boy beside me got up, staggered to the wall, and began to climb up to the narrow window. He moved with the agility of a cat, using the bench and then my thigh as a ladder. He stood on the windowsill, tried the window lock, opened the window partway, then slammed it shut again. The windowsill was barely wide enough to accommodate his tiny feet. I raised my hands behind him in case he tumbled backward but was careful not to touch him for fear I might provoke his ire and suffer a slap.

I knew that this was not a formal class, that it was just a forty-five-minute pre-lunch period in which Kyumi had offered to share his linguistic and Braille skills with the beginners, but things seemed to me to be getting out of hand, and I had the sense that I was some-how the cause of the chaos. Apparently sensing the same thing, Kyumi walked around the end of the table and marched toward me. "Rose," he said with some consternation, "I am happy to help you learn Tibet-an alphabet, but...please, you must *study*."

"Yes, of course," I said. "I'm very sorry for interrupting you."

"No problem, Rose. But *please* listen."

"Yes, Kyumi, I certainly will."

"Good. And after this I teach them English alphabet such as *A, B, C, D*."

Kyumi had not got much farther in the lesson before he put his hand to his crotch and announced to the room that he had to pee. He informed us that he would go out of the room briefly, that he would promptly return, and that we should all carry on with our work without interruptions or delay. He ran to the door, swung it open, and dashed down the hallway.

The class members applied themselves to their work. Mingmar, sitting cross-legged on the table, seemed at a loss for what to do now. She drummed her fingertips on her lips, as if searching for ideas. Remembering the Monk, she scooted down and lit into him again, forcing his hands onto the table where she thought his page of Braille lay. The page, however, had fluttered to the floor. When I told her this, she leaped off the table, fell to her hands and knees, and began patting the floor around the Monk's chair until she found it. She jumped back onto the table, put the page before the Monk, and spoke to him with good-natured urgency, entreating him to try. The Monk was a year or two older than Mingmar and almost twice her size, yet he allowed her to manipulate his hands on the page. Gradually, as he listened to the zeal in her piping voice and felt her small jabs of encouragement on his upper arm, the corners of his mouth began to show the faintest trace of a smile. *"Ka,"* he said, because what choice did he really have?

Satisfied that the Monk was on his way, Mingmar jumped off the table and ran into the kitchen singing a song in Chinese. Kyumi returned from the toilet and began to read aloud a list of words from a page of Braille. Minutes passed. We listened and learned. At one point Kyumi stood behind me, said a word in Tibetan, then said, "Rose, in English this word means 'screet.' Do you like screet?"

I twisted around in my seat to look at him. "Screet? I don't think we have such a word in English."

"Yes, yes," he said, "it is this!" He raised his fingers to his lips and pretended to puff on an imaginary cigarette. "It smells nice and there is smoke."

"*Cigarette,* you mean?"

"Yes. I like to smoke screet. Do you like?"

"No, I don't smoke."

"And I like to fight." Kyumi continued to drag on the nonexistent cigarette with one hand and made a threatening fist with the other.

"You like smoking and fighting?"

He crossed his arms in a stance of defiance. "Yes. I like. And tomorrow I fight all China."

"You're going to fight all of China? Why?"

"I don't like China. I want to kill all China. Because one Chinese man, he say to me, 'Kyumi, I kill you.'"

"A Chinese person said that to you?"

He put his hands on his hips, unafraid. "Chinese want to kill all Tibet. So I want to kill all China. Rose, do you fight China?"

With his right hand, Kyumi grasped his own left wrist and began to flap his left hand rapidly up and down in the air; it fluttered like a cotton dishrag. Kyumi was so small, I could probably have hoisted him up onto my shoulders and carried him half a mile or so without tiring. I looked at the jug ears, the amusing round pink face, the fluttering hands—he was a fussy bundle of nerves and totally blind, but he was extremely intelligent and confident enough to believe that he could take on all of China with his fists in the air and a cigarette dangling from his ruby-red lips.

"I have no reason to fight the Chinese," I said, "and fighting is not a good way to solve problems anyway."

Determining, I think, that I was not only disruptive but an irredeemable dummy and a bit of a bore, Kyumi moved away to the far end of the table and began collecting the Braille sheets. "Time for lunch now," he said.

Other children had begun to come into the dining room, throwing their book bags into a corner and spearing their white canes into the cane box. I had noticed a schedule on the wall outside the dining room indicating what child was assigned to what communal task on which day. There was a cleaning schedule, a dishwashing schedule, a serving schedule. A sixteen-year-old boy named Ngudup came into the dining room with a bunch of spoons in his hand and began laying them out on the tables. Ngudup had hollow eyes, shaggy black hair, and heavy eyebrows. He was extremely gangly. The sleeve of his jacket was split at the seam, and his trousers were cinched around his narrow waist with a stiff leather belt. Ngudup was one of the older students in the school; I could see the faint shadow of a mustache beginning to present itself on his upper lip. Ngudup had spent the first eleven years of his life locked in a small dark room.

The children found seats on the benches; there was some jostling for space, some clashing of elbows, and one or two of them accidentally sat down in other children's laps. Once they were settled, the cook and two of the older students began serving the food—rice, vegetables, and yak meat—in metal bowls. They sat with their bowls before them, waiting patiently until everyone was seated and served. Finally, they all raised their bowls off the table in a worshipful way and began singing a Tibetan prayer that involved a lot of *om-om-om*-ing. Then the bowls were returned to the tabletop and they dug in with their spoons. They ate in silence, leaning forward with their mouths very close to the edge of the bowls. Some of the smaller ones lifted the bowls to their lips and shoveled the food directly into their mouths. They were very small and thin, and their clothes, obviously secondhand donations, were ill-fitting, but they seemed very much at ease and at home here. A few of them spilled food on the table, then unwittingly rested their sleeves in it. Some rice and vegetables landed on the floor, but overall the meal was surprisingly tidy. And when they finished, they either brought their bowls to the kitchen for more or carried them to the sink to be washed.

I sat in the dining room until the last child, Dolma, had finished her lunch. Somehow Dolma knew that I was still sitting at the end of the table. She made her way to me, blinked her strange blind eyes at the sky that was framed by the windows beside me, and confessed to me that she did not like her own name. She wanted a different name. Did I have any ideas for a better name for her? I was so surprised by the request that I said too quickly, "How about Shirley?" Why I said this, I do not know. I have never liked the name Shirley. As soon as I said it, I regretted it. A girl from a warrior tribe such as hers deserved something a bit more sturdy and dignified. But it was too late—she seized on Shirley with great glee, and when she repeated it, it sounded very much like a Chinese name. Dolma headed out the door of the dining room smiling and blinking and announcing proudly to no one, "I am Shirley!" I forgave myself with the thought that "I am Shirley" was, at the very least, a step up from "I am a witch."

As I was getting up to attend the next scheduled class, Ngudup came back into the dining room with a mop in his hands and began cleaning the floor. He seemed to know the exact location of all the furniture in the room. He mopped swiftly and smoothly beneath the tables and benches, never bumping into anything and not missing any sections of the floor, and all the while he hummed a tune steadily under his breath. For a few moments, when he mopped the floor in front of the full-length mirror, his figure was reflected in such a way that he appeared to be a pair of people mopping in graceful tandem. He could have had no idea that his image was being duplicated like this. As I walked by him to leave the room I realized that the song he was humming was the Turtles' 1960s hit "Happy Together." Sensing that I was passing near him, Ngudup raised his head and stopped humming. It seemed rude to go by without saying anything, especially as he could not have known who exactly was in the room with him, a situation I would find vexing and unpleasant were I to find myself in his position.

I said hello to him, and he smiled and nodded his head at the sound of my voice but was too shy to say anything in return and continued pushing his mop.

As I was going down the hallway, I saw Kyila, the nineteen-year-old girl who would soon be going to England, coming toward me from the opposite direction. I had spoken to her only once since I'd arrived at the school, but as she passed me, she said, "Hi, Rose." Surprised, I stopped her and asked how she knew it was me.

She said matter-of-factly but politely, "Oh, smell."

"Do I smell?"

She laughed. "Well, not in a bad way. But you smell...different from the other people."

I was fascinated and eager to know what it was that she smelled. "What is it?" I said. "What is the smell?"

The girl stepped closer. She paused a minute, thinking. "The hair, maybe? Shampoo, maybe. Or soap."

The hallway was dark. I tried my best to smell the girl from the same distance that she was smelling me. I smelled nothing but the lingering aromas of lunch drifting down from the kitchen. I knew there was no way that I would be able to tell one individual in the school from another just by smell, even if I stayed here a month. No way in the world. But why was that? If this girl could do it—even though it seemed extremely odd to me that she could—shouldn't I be able to learn to do it? After all, I could identify people on the telephone just by their voices. I could identify foods just by tasting them. I might even be able to recognize a familiar face just by feeling it, though that would be a difficult task if I hadn't seen the person in a long time and wasn't expecting him to show up beside me.

As I was crossing the courtyard to the classroom building it came to me that even before I had opened my mouth in the dining room, Ngudup most probably had known that it was I who was in the room with him and no other person. It began to dawn on me then that it is very difficult to hide from a blind person, and that if you think you can take advantage of another person's sightlessness, you are probably in for a surprise. It was a revelation I would be reminded of countless times over the next few years.

The next class I attended was a formal English class in which some of the older students practiced their English Braille typing. The students sat at small individual desks of the sort you'd see in any grade school. The desks had probably once been arranged in regular rows, but now they were slightly scattered and aslant of one another, having been repeatedly knocked into. The more experienced among the students used Braille typewriters; the others used Braille slates—flat boards with Braille templates cut into them. The slate was worked with a thing called a stylus, a knob roughly the shape of a champagne cork with a blunt needle at the end of it; with the needle, the student punched the dots of the Braille letters through the template and into the paper below it. There was a gentle tapping sound on the desks, like light rain on a rooftop, as they worked their pins.

The teacher, a young blind woman named Pema, sat at a large table at the front of the class reciting lines for the students to type out. I sat at a small desk beside hers. The windows of the classroom, several of which were open, faced a public street. The occasional sound of drilling drifted up from a construction site nearby. Pema wore her hair in a long ponytail tied with a pink ribbon. The older girls in the class sat at the back of the room, working hard, glowering at the ceiling as they thought, or lowering their heads intently to their machines. They had plump faces and were shy and diligent, and they too wore their hair in long ponytails tied with brightly colored ribbons. In their early teens, they were more focused than the younger girls, calmer, and seemed intent on getting on with their learning. They ticked out Braille words with their typewriters, now and then feeling the words on the page to make sure they had formed them correctly. Occasionally they reached over and felt each other's pages, squinting critically, consulting one another in Tibetan about an English word. Once in a while, a page would jam in the typewriter, and then the girl would suck air through her teeth with frustration and wrestle the page free, her fingers flying over the metal components of the machine. Once the page was loosened, the girl felt its surface carefully to make sure the raised type hadn't been damaged.

The teacher asked individual students to translate into English a line or a phrase that she read out in Tibetan, and when the student answered correctly, the entire class applauded. She said something in Tibetan, and a girl at the back of the room stood up and replied, "Food is good." That met with a round of applause. Another girl in the front row jumped up uninvited and improved upon the answer by shouting, "Food is dee-licious!" Then she knocked on the wall for emphasis and added, accurately but quite off the script, "This is a wall!," and sat back down. The girl's name, I knew, was Sangmu. She had the unbecoming bowl-like haircut of a medieval serf. Her eyes were whitish blue with cataracts, like the eyes of an aging dog, and now and then they jittered up and down in their sockets with an almost electronic rapidity. I later learned that while Sangmu was living with her family in a small remote village, her father used to beat her repeatedly, irked no doubt by her blindness and her jittering eyes.

The teacher recited another phrase, and the entire class said in unison, "My bicycle is old!"

Sangmu stood up again and in a correcting way repeated the sentence with perfect clarity—"My! Bicycle! Is! Old!"—showing them all how proper English should sound. She wore a rough brown checkered jacket that looked as though it had been made from an old woolen blanket. Her red corduroy trousers had Mickey Mouse embroidered on one leg. On her wrist was a tin bracelet, and beside her chair lay a Mickey Mouse book bag of pink and blue. (Looking around, I realized that Mickey Mouse was represented seven or eight times in the room, on backpacks and jackets and trouser pockets.) It quickly became evident that Sangmu was the most confident English speaker in the class—when the teacher called out a phrase, she had finished translating it before anyone else had even begun. "Small nose! Big tree! Nice car! Where is the h-o-s-p-i-t-a-l?" Like many of the students, she had the distinctly Tibetan habit of spelling out the words she heard as a way of learning and remembering them. She seemed a bit bored and fidgeted ceaselessly at her desk, tearing a piece of paper off her Braille page and twisting it into a slender corkscrew shape that she then fitted carefully up her nose in a testing way. The test made her sneeze rapidly three times in a row, delicate little sneezes that sounded like a match being struck repeatedly. She put her head on her desk, felt the wall, picked up a baseball cap that had been lying on her desk and put it on her head, took it off again, and scribbled on the wall with a fingernail. She pulled something out of her jacket pocket, held it to her nose, and sniffed at it several times. It was a metal bottle cap that obviously still retained the pleasant scent of whatever soft drink it had once contained. I understood by now that blind children were always searching for any kind of sensory stimulation for entertainment—sound, smell, touch, and motion. Sangmu's fidgeting seemed to express innate optimism, an enthusiasm about simply being alive. Finally she lowered her head and returned her hands resignedly to her stylus.

The teacher called on a girl in the second row. The girl stood up. She had a pigtail protruding horizontally from behind each ear, and abnormally large eyes that were almost solid black in color and opaque as stones. There was next to no differentiation in the pigment of her dark brown eyeball—no discernible iris or pupil and very little white. They brought to mind the eyes of a horse. Her name was Dechen, and despite the strange eyes she was extremely pretty, with full red lips and pink cheeks and long black lashes. Dechen was shy and spoke her assigned sentence haltingly. "Heez coawat eeez beeeg." When the students applauded, Dechen sank back into her seat and put her head on her desk in mortification, and the two pigtails angled up like the handlebars on a tricycle.

Sangmu stood up and repeated Dechen's sentence clearly: "His! Coat! Is! Big!" The teacher said something brisk to Sangmu in Tibetan, and Sangmu sat down again, grinning hugely and swinging her feet beneath her chair, seemingly delighted at having been told to pipe down. She was so eager for new experiences that even a dressing-down from the teacher was a welcome excitement.

An old man with a very wrinkled face and a battered fedora perched on his head at a rakish slant appeared at one of the open windows. He stared into the room with a look of complete puzzlement, trying to make sense of what was going on here. A boy with the anxious face of Peter Lorre stood up and said, "I sell you!"

Sangmu could not contain herself. Without even bothering to stand she twisted around in her seat and cried, "No! That is wrong. You must say, 'I *see* you.'"

Chagrined at his mistake, the boy swiped his hand down the length of his own face, as if to erase it. He accepted Sangmu's correction. "I *see* you."

"But you *cannot* see me!" Sangmu cried with great mirth.

A chubby boy behind her with a pair of worn bedroom slippers on his feet offered suddenly, "I can see a little with this eye but not with this one."

"Because you are blind!" Sangmu said, as though his blindness were cause for celebration. "*We* are blind," she added, and the other students laughed in proud agreement.

Why were they laughing? That was the question constantly at the back of my mind as I made my way among the students of Braille

Without Borders. Why had so many said to me "I am happy I'm blind"? Why were they happy and laughing, eager to do their studies, eager to teach one another? Why weren't they all brooding and languishing like the poor little Monk or crying out, *Why me, God?* Plenty of them had started life with sight and then gradually lost it, so they were at least vaguely aware of what they were missing. Beggars and others who could not afford to be choosers had spat at them and thrown stones at them, ridiculed and spurned them. Some of them had been abandoned by their families, some beaten, some tied to furniture. Where did the cheerfulness come from? Was it simply that they had, for the first time, found other children like themselves? Was it that they had, purely by chance, been found by someone who saw beneath the surface of them, who knew that behind their dull eyes, a whole universe of thought was simmering, waiting to be given a chance?

The old man in the window squinted and stared, leaning on the windowsill with both arms, his mouth hanging open in interest and absorption. He looked somehow mistrustful of the sound of this foreign language coming from people so young. Because the students were facing away from him, he couldn't see that they were blind. He called something to the teacher across the students' dark heads. The teacher, who could not see him, ignored him, and so he harrumphed and went away.

I was the only person in the room who could see that the students in this classroom were blind. Most of them looked blind, with eyes that were damaged or skewed or just plain didn't open. Most of them had no idea what their classmates looked like; most would not know that Sangmu's eyes jittered or that Dechen's eyes were like a horse's or that Ngudup's eyes were sunken or that Mingmar's eyes were slits. Most of them could not see Mickey Mouse adorning their clothing and accessories, raring to go with his white-gloved hand raised in a convivial wave to the world at large and his pink tongue annoyingly visible in his perpetually smiling mouth. Most of them could not see the teacher's ponytail or the shiny orange walls of their classroom. Most of them could not see me and knew who I was only by the sound of my voice or the smell of my shampoo.

"Hospital is on the left!"

"M-i-n-u-t-e-s!"

The classroom ticked with the sound of the Braille machines. The teacher read out more sentences.

"Go straight then left to the hospital," said a girl whose blind eyes were hopelessly crossed. (This girl had asked Sabriye soon after her arrival at the school, "Why is it that the children in my village throw stones at me, but everyone here is nice to me?")

Kalden, a grinning snaggletoothed boy with a big head, a gnomish face, and a red scarf tied around his neck, stood up and said, "He buys a gun." Kalden's eyes were obscured by the cloudy white film of cataracts, a common affliction here.

Someone at the back of the room made the sound of a gun, and the class collapsed in giggles.

"This is my foot."

"This is my eyes."

"Y-o-u-r mother is a bye!"

"No!" Sangmu cried. "Your m-o-t-h-e-r is a *girl*."

At the end of the class the teacher stood up and began gathering her books. Some of the older students made their way to her desk and handed her the Braille pages they had typed. Then some returned to their desks and continued working. None of the students seemed in a great hurry to leave the classroom. A few of them wandered close to where I was sitting and, realizing that I was there, began to question me and investigate my possessions. Kalden approached, bumped into my desk, found my hand, and held on to it. The boy who looked like Peter Lorre came and took my pen out of my other hand and pretended to write on the desk with it. He was wearing a jean jacket with embroidery on the breast that depicted a man playing tennis; beneath the man was written *WE R'E # 1!* Sangmu came over and ran her hands over my little desk. When she found my notebook, she said, "What is this?"

"That is my notebook," I said.

"For what?"

"For writing down ideas."

Sangmu smiled, opened the notebook, lifted it to her blind eyes, and pretended to read what I had written: "'Sangmu is a very, very good girl!'" That notion cast her into a seizure of laughter.

# The Neglected Senses

At Braille Without Borders, you learn quickly not to stand idly in doorways or on staircases or in narrow hallways, for the consequence is that eventually somebody blind will slam into you. In settings familiar to the blind, the unobstructed navigability of transitional passageways is something they quite reasonably take for granted. A doorway exists solely to be passed through, a staircase solely to be ascended or descended, a hallway solely to be traversed on the way from one room to another. Unable to see that a two-hundred-pound man is sitting in the middle of a staircase, a pack of blind students will most likely fail to anticipate his anomalous presence and fall headlong over him as they attempt to skip down the stairs. The students at BWB race around their school, sprinting down the hallways, turning corners crisply at five miles per hour, skirting tables and chairs, opening doors without groping for the knobs, reaching for objects on shelves with surprising precision. They kick soccer balls, rearrange furniture, zip their own zippers, throw things and catch things (yes, sometimes they miss the catch and the things end up hitting them in the face), fill their own soup bowls, go for walks downtown alone, make purchases without getting shortchanged. They know their realm so well that after a few days at the school, I began to forget that they were blind and would not have been entirely surprised to find a blind child successfully juggling three apples or using the banister as a balance beam. I realized that those who had some vision actually moved more hesitantly than those who were completely blind. The slightly sighted, still depending on their weakened eyes, had to take time to make out what they were seeing—to locate a doorknob, for example—and sometimes they thought they could see where they were going but miscalculated and ended up crashing into tables or posts. Also, those who could see a bit were more distractible than those who couldn't see at all, and they occasionally tried to read their Braille with whatever sight they had left, holding the embossed pages an inch from their eyes, a habit that Paul and Sabriye adamantly discouraged, because it taxes whatever vision remains and because it is much less efficient than tactile reading.

I was surprised by the ease and harmony the blind students had with their physical realm and was eager enough to understand it that at Sabriye's suggestion I agreed to let myself be blindfolded and led through the streets of Lhasa by two blind teenage girls, Choden and Yangchen.

The girls and I set off from the school and as soon as we crossed the big boulevard, Chingdol Dong Lu, I took a blindfold out of my pocket. Yangchen and Choden stood on either side of me, waiting expectantly, holding their white canes before them, clearly amused by the challenge. Yangchen, a shy, round-faced, cross-eyed sixteen-year-old with her hair in a ponytail, was completely blind in one eye and saw only faint impressions of light with the other. She wore a baseball cap, clodhopper boots, a plaid flannel shirt buttoned up to the throat, denim trousers, and a jean jacket. Yangchen's perpetually crossed eyes gave her the appearance of slapstick confusion. I came to learn, however, that Yangchen was a level-headed, sober, practical girl and possessed of considerable poise. Choden, a year younger than Yangchen, was pink-cheeked and ever smiling. She too wore a ponytail, plaid flannel shirt, denim jacket and pants, baseball cap, and hiking boots. Side by side in their rough-and-ready attire, the girls brought to mind a pair of lumberjacks ready to chop their way through a forest. Choden's eyes were pinched shut most of the time, but her left eye occasionally opened and seemed to range around in its orbit taking in some light and color.

The girls' blindness, their white canes, and my foreign presence with them had drawn a group of onlookers on the city sidewalk. As I pulled the blindfold over my eyes, I said to the girls, "We have a lot of people looking at us."

Excited and embarrassed, they hooted "Heeoo!" into their fingertips.

"And," I added, "one of the people looking at us is a tall Chinese policeman with a gun."

To that dire piece of information they responded with a moment of shocked silence. And then they lowered their heads and muttered gravely, "Tchah!"

"But," I said, "never mind the people. I have put the blindfold on and cannot see them anymore. I am now putting my sunglasses on over the blindfold so that I can see even less."

"Good," Yangchen said. "Now you are blind?"

My eyes were sufficiently bound that I could see nothing at all— no light, no forms, nothing. The bright and varied colors of the buildings of Lhasa had disappeared, and I was presented with nothing but the backs of my own eyelids onto which my heartbeat was projected in rhythmic flashes of orange. In the high altitude and resultant low atmospheric pressure of Lhasa, I was often aware that my heart was struggling to do its job. Nowhere else in the world had I been so conscious of my own pulse. At night when I lay in bed, my heart pounded in my chest, ears, and eyes and I felt short of breath to the point that I slept with my mouth open and occasionally woke up feeling that I might actually be suffocating, whereupon I had to get up and walk around my enormous hotel room.* Sometimes I even had to stand by an open window and inhale deeply (which only gave me the comforting *illusion* that I was getting more air when of course the reality was that the atmospheric pressure outside the room was exactly the same as it was inside it) until the suffocating feeling passed.

"I can't see a thing, I assure you," I said. "Now, listen, girls, you won't let me get lost in Lhasa, will you? You know I don't speak Tibetan."

With a hint of gloating pleasure Choden said, "Yah. We know it." Then she took my hand and thrust her white cane into it.

"Oh, am I taking a cane too?"

Yangchen, the older of the two, interjected nervously, "Cane? Well, no. Maybe no cane. Choden must have her own cane. Otherwise she can lose her road."

I passed the cane clumsily back to Choden. "Take your cane, Choden. God forbid you should lose your road while you're leading me."

The girls positioned themselves on either side of me, hooked their arms through mine, and we headed up the street. Immediately I had the sensation that the ground beneath my feet was tilting. Sound seemed to become louder, smells became stronger, and the breeze on my face felt more forceful and distracting. I tripped on a raised lip of pavement, and the girls quickly tightened their grip on my elbows to keep me from falling. The dragging clicking of one of the canes on the pavement sounded for all the world like the jittering ball in a spinning roulette wheel. I asked Choden if it was her cane that was making all that noise.

"Yah. Very nizey is my cane." Compelled to imitate the gravelly sound of her cane, Choden said with relish, "Zaaaarrrrr!"

---

*The room, like every other room in the hotel, was roughly the size of a conference room in Beijing's Great Hall of the People. This, I had decided, was a concession to the Tibetan comfort and familiarity with vast open spaces.

Sensing that I was nervous, Yangchen said, "Rose, how you are feeling?"

"Well, I'm not really afraid," I said, "but I feel as though I'm in a boat that's moving. You know that feeling when you're in a boat and the water is moving beneath you and you're a little bit unsteady on your feet?"

"Oh, yah, I know it! Funny," Choden said. "You are a little bit nervous, is that right, Rose?"

I confessed that I was indeed a little bit nervous.

This seemed to please Choden. "Oh, ha!" she said, audibly smiling.

"Have you ever been in a boat?" I asked her.

"No, I never."

"Well, then how can you say you know how it feels?"

"Oh, ha! You are right."

"Tell me, girls, how do you feel? Does the ground feel steady to you?"

"Yah," Yangchen said, "is always steady. No problem. And now we must turn left."

"How do you know that?"

"Because the sound of many televisions."

Until Yangchen mentioned it, I had not noticed the sound of many televisions. I had vaguely heard some background noise beyond us, an insignificant presence at the periphery of my attention, but distracted by my nervousness, I had not identified it. Now, focusing on it, I realized that the sound of many televisions was quite loud; riotous, in fact— it was that unmistakably tinny television sound, a counterfeit, thinner version of firsthand sound. What I was hearing was the many-times-multiplied voices of two people having a tense dialogue in Chinese; they spoke with the razor-sharp accent of Beijing. And then I heard rapid gunfire; filtered and squeezed through the many televisions, the gunfire sounded feeble and fake, like plastic popguns in a penny arcade. I was disturbed that I hadn't noticed these sounds from a distance.

"That is men always selling televisions in a shop," Yangchen said. "Sometimes it is war films. When we hear the televisions, we know we must turn left."

It was a matter of familiarity, then, a recognizable constant in the girls' journey into the city.

We carried on at an alarmingly brisk pace. I expected at any moment to crack my forehead on a lamppost or go plummeting into an open manhole. I felt terribly vulnerable and had to fight the impulse to lift the blindfold off my face. As I walked I realized that I was holding my chin much higher in the air than I normally would, the way I do when I'm swimming and trying to keep my head dry, and each step I took had the same quality of awkward anticipation as those last few exploratory, drop-footed steps taken toward the bottom of a staircase one is descending in the pitch-dark. I couldn't help lifting my hands in front of me in self-defense, like a pathetic caricature of a blind person. Linked at the elbows with the two girls, I found it difficult to lift my hands; nevertheless, I kept trying to lift them, and Yangchen kept gently pressing them down to show me I had nothing to fear.

"I shouldn't lift my hands, Yangchen?" I said.

"Umm. Maybe it is better to trust," Yangchen said. She was much too patient and polite a girl to just come out and say *No, you shouldn't*.

"Girls," I said, "I wouldn't be able to do this alone."

"You would be afraid?" Choden said.

"I would be very afraid."

"Oh, ha," Choden said.

"Do not be afraid," Yangchen said. "We are watching you."

All the blind students spoke this way— *We are watching you. Nice to see you. See you again. Please let me see that book.* For them, the vocabulary of vision was metaphorical, a symbolic representation of human connection, interest, and concern.

The girls coaxed me forward with their slender arms, never breaking their stride. I heard passing voices speaking Tibetan and Chinese, the sound of a small spluttering engine like that of a generator or an idling motorbike, the distant shrieks of children, a horn that sounded like a loud fart, something metallic scraping briefly on the pavement behind us, someone sneezing richly nearby, and all the while Choden's noisy cane rattling along in front of us like a yapping little dog leading the way.

Yangchen had a habit of humming as she walked. Each time she spoke, she had to interrupt her own humming, putting it on hold until there was silence between us again, whereupon she would resume the tune approximately where she had left off. I asked the girls how long they had been blind; both said from a very young age. I asked them what they had been doing before they came to Braille Without Borders in Lhasa.

Yangchen said, "I was only at home. Just praying something and helping my mother."

Choden said, "I'm too home. Praying and helping."

"Were there any other blind kids where you lived?"

"My country don't have blind kids," Choden said. "Only me."

"Not my country either," Yangchen said.

I knew that what they meant by "my country" were the villages they had come from, small mountain hamlets with mud-brick houses, muttering flocks of chickens, some goats, shaggy yaks with matted hair, and little else but the biggest sky in the world, an all-engulfing sunlight, and a distant backdrop of seriously jagged snowcapped mountains.

Yangchen informed me out of the blue that her father died when she was young and that her mother was, at present, dying. I was so taken aback that I couldn't bring myself to ask what her mother was dying of. Prompted by the mention of parents, Choden said, "My mother was pregnant with me, and a cow kick her in the stomach one time, and so that is why I got blind."

I thought about the physics of this. "Are you sure that's why you're blind, Choden?" I said.

"Yah. Sure," she said cheerfully, and she gave my arm a little squeeze, as if to assure me that it really was quite all right to have the future of your eyesight mystically predetermined by a wayward, mud-encrusted cow's hoof even before you were born. Like most Tibetans, the blind students were deeply conscious of reincarnation and karmic retribution. The widespread Tibetan impulse to go to the temple and pray was not just an effort to achieve a higher spirituality but also a warding-off of the malign and omnipresent supernatural forces believed to be pressing upon each individual's life and destiny.

I asked the girls if they still prayed now that they were in Lhasa. Yes, every morning at seven they went to the temple to pray. What exactly were they praying for? For the goodness, they said, and good things and to make up for sins.

What kind of sins?

There was a silence while they thought about this. "Mmm, sometimes we broke some things at school," Choden said.

What things?

"Everythings! Braille machines and desks and—"

"And windows," Yangchen interjected.

"Because we cannot see and we make an accident sometimes."

I pointed out that these were not sins but forgivable mistakes. They thought about it, then agreed with me. A long silence followed while they searched their souls for real and purposive sins. I knew that the silence was due not to their reluctance to tell me their sins but to their inability to find anything really worthy to confess.

"Okay," I said, "never mind the sins."

"And anyway now we go right," Yangchen said, gently steering me with her arm.

"How do you know that?"

"You feel the ground got different here under your feet?"

I had felt nothing. But now that Yangchen had brought it to my attention, I realized that the ground we were walking on was very uneven. When I told the girls that I had felt nothing different, that the ground had seemed to me to be always uneven, they stopped, turned me around, and took me back to the start of the street.

"Rose, now we show you. You must go and feel the street here." Yangchen tapped my shin firmly with her cane to indicate that I should try the street out with my foot; the gesture was surprisingly authoritative. It was also intimate in the way the gestures of a good teacher often are. "You feel how it feels."

I smeared the soles of my shoes around. "It feels smooth, like concrete pavement."

"Yah, smooth. Now come and you walk." We walked ten paces on the smooth pavement and then, very abruptly, the pavement changed and became something like cobblestone or roughly hewn brick. The first time around, I hadn't registered the change, which astonished me, because the contrast was in fact sudden and marked. I had simply not been paying attention to what was under my feet. Why would I? When one is in the habit of anticipating the path ahead by sight, one rarely makes conscious note of or even actually *feels* in any lasting way the texture of that path.*

"When we feel the ground coming different under our feet, we know where we find ourselves," Yangchen said.

---

*How well do you know the sidewalk on your own street? You think you know it, but put on a blindfold and walk around on it and you'll likely find that you don't know your sidewalk at all. You'll find cracks and grooves, trees, hydrants, and signposts that are unfamiliar to you because you never truly noticed them. Walk face-first into one of those trees and you'll never again forget that it's there. Samuel Clemens, an avid champion of Helen Keller, stated firmly to a skeptical friend, "Blindness is an exciting business...if you don't believe it, get up some dark night on the wrong side of your bed when the house is on fire and try to find the door."

"Do you know when a person is walking close to you?"

"Yes, because we can hear them. And also sometimes can smell them. And also our cane can describe to us whatever is near us."

I told the girls their English was quite good and asked them if they were continuing to study the language.

"Yah. Now we are learning how to speak in a restaurant," Yangchen said.

I wasn't sure what she meant by that. By way of explanation, Choden said in the tone of an extremely nervous, extremely unctuous waitress, "Hello, madam. You are so very welcome. Good evening, can I help you, please? What would you like to please eat?"

In the voice of a customer who had memorized the entire menu and was bored stiff by it, Yangchen responded, "Yes, please. I would like to have please one yak s-t-e-a-k."

"Oh, very fine," Choden said. "Please, how would you like your yak s-t-e-a-k to be cooked?"

"I would like to have my yak steak to be cooked m-e-d-i-u-m rare, please."

"What would you please like to drink, please? Would you like to drink some of coffee?"

"Please," Yangchen said, "I would like a bottle of white w-i-n-d."

"Yangchen," I said, "w-i-n-d spells *wind*. A bottle of white wind would be something very rare, if not completely impossible."

Yangchen stopped in her tracks and positively guffawed at her mistake. "Oh, ha-ha-ha! No! Please, a bottle of white wine, please, I mean."

I told the girls that it was not necessary for them to use the word *please* every time they opened their mouths in a restaurant.

"No?"

"No. Once or twice is really enough. Otherwise you will become quite annoying."

"What does it mean, *annoying*?" Yangchen asked.

I explained that being annoying meant that soon enough the person you were serving in the restaurant would have a strong desire to slap you. Immediately they understood. True to Tibetan form, the girls did not let the word *annoying* go by without asking me how to spell it.

We walked on, listening to the sounds passing by—hammering, a squeaky wheel, birds chittering, voices speaking in Chinese and Tibetan, a horn being blown—and suddenly at my right shoulder, Yangchen interrupted her humming to ask me, "Rose, what is your hoppy?"

This question always surprises me and makes me uneasy, perhaps because I never have a plausible-sounding answer to the question. If a hobby is something one pursues purely for pleasure, then reading the Greek-English dictionary and another excellent book called *600 Modern Greek Verbs: Fully Conjugated in All the Tenses* is my hobby. I can become engrossed in those books so deeply—one word leading to another—that I fail to notice an entire hour passing. But how to explain this in an offhand way to a person you don't know well? As a hobby, it sounds not only pointless and dull but pretentious and pedantic as well. I have no desire to explain it. Anything I could truly claim as a hobby I am always reluctant to reveal. And the very concept of the hobby strikes me as too parochial, too specific, by definition too distinctly separate from life's main activities.

I told Yangchen that in general I liked rowing a boat, riding a bicycle, and making things out of wood—all the activities I liked that seemed to need no explanation or defense.

Yangchen said, "I like sing a song and learn some song and I also like rotten."

"Rotten? What's that?"

"Rotten. Rotten."

"Can you spell the word for me?"

"I cannot."

Choden tried to spell it for her. "Rot. R-o-t. R-o-t-e-n."

"Well, I hear what you're saying, but I'm not sure what you mean by it," I said. "*Rotten* is an adjective. It cannot be a hobby."

"Tchah! I am wrong." Yangchen tittered and laid the side of her face against my upper arm, half in embarrassment and half in apology.

I felt a soft breeze on my cheek. "Now it's a little windy," I said.

"Windy, yah."

"How come all of a sudden?" I guessed the answer. "Are we out of the closed street and in an open place?"

"You are right," Yangchen said. "We are in open and it is wind and there is a cloud."

"How do you know there's a cloud?"

"I do not feel the sun on my nose."

"I didn't notice that," I said.

"Oh, ha," Choden said.

By now I had learned that this was Choden's default response. When she didn't know what to say but wanted to maintain active participation in the conversation, she said encouragingly, *Oh, ha.*

I heard the sound of water splashing, like a hose or a downspout pouring onto a pavement. "Where is that splashing water coming from?" I said.

"Not water," Yangchen said. "That noise is frying of dumplings. Here is a small restaurant in the street."

Before long I heard the crashing sound of thunder.

"No," Choden said. "Not thunder. That is only the door of the marketplace. They are closing it. It makes a big noise."

The closing door sounded so much like thunder that I wanted to pull off my blindfold and look around to be sure that Choden wasn't tricking me. I asked Choden if she was sure it wasn't thunder.

"Yah, Rose, sure. Don't worry."

"Now I smell gasoline," I said.

"No. That is shoes smell."

"What?"

"Shoes smell. *Hongo*." The two girls conferred in Tibetan, trying to figure out how to explain to me what I was smelling. "It is the smell of shoes. They are selling the shoes here in the street."

I heard birdsong coming from somewhere behind us, a clear wandering whistle like that of a robin. I remarked on it, and Choden said, "No, it is not a bird. It is..." She said something to Yangchen in Tibetan, looking again for a word.

"Alarm. It is the alarm for a car in case a person tries to steal it."

They knew everything about their city. They knew what everything was and where it was and how it sounded and smelled and felt. They knew it by heart and with their eyes closed. It seemed to me that they knew the city every bit as well as its sighted residents, and I was beginning to wonder whether I too couldn't benefit from knowing my environment from this different perspective.

"Now the cloud went and the sun came shining," Yangchen said, and as soon as she said it I felt the sun on my head.

"Now we turn left," Choden said.

"How do you know we turn left?"

"We smell the incense. That smells very nice. It means we are nearly in Jokhang Temple."

The moment Choden mentioned it, the air was full of the smell of incense. Again, I hadn't noticed it until she alerted me to it. The girls were always one step ahead of me, maybe two. I had detected very little of what was taking place around me on this walk, perhaps because I was nervous and disoriented, but also because I was so used to navigating with my eyes that my other senses, relative to the senses of the blind girls, were atrophied. I stumbled along uncomfortably, feeling out of control and disliking that I was so slow in grasping and noticing what they noticed.

Sight is a slick and overbearing autocrat, trumpeting its prodigal knowledge and perceptions so forcefully that it drowns out the other, subtler senses. We go through our day semi-oblivious to a whole range of sensory information because we are distracted and enslaved by our eyes. Taste, touch, smell, and hearing can hardly get a word in edgewise to the brain. Those of us who have sight do not realize that our experience of life and the world is overpowered by our vision. In this sense, we too are handicapped. I began to envy Choden's and Yangchen's skills a little. In their presence, I saw that I had been missing a great deal of what was happening in my daily life, and I realized that it was not the blind person's deficiency that was drawing me into this subject but the revelation of my own.*

Now that the girls had drawn it to my attention, the smell of incense was very strong. It was sweet and flowery, cloying as cheap perfume. I sensed there were many people near us now. I heard soft voices, tinkling bells, and a horn being blown on a low note. I knew where we were and what was taking place, because I had been here a few days before. Jokhang Temple, located in Barkhor Square in the center of Lhasa, is the most sacred temple in Tibet. Throngs of Buddhist pilgrims come from all over the country to worship here. I knew (because I had seen it) that in front of the Jokhang Temple, where the girls and I were now sightlessly standing, there were so many pilgrims prostrating themselves that the square looked like a refugee encampment. There had been so much to look at when I was last here—multicolored, fantastical, and bizarre—that I hadn't really noticed the smell of incense, even though it burned in great quantities in a kind of specially con-

---

*Of this phenomenon Jacques Lusseyran wrote, "Sight is a miraculous instrument offering us all the riches of physical life. But we get nothing in this world without paying for it, and in return for all the benefits that sight brings we are forced to give up others whose existence we don't even suspect."

structed pear-shaped chimney that looked roughly a thousand years old and that sent great gouts of bluish smoke billowing into the air in front of the temple.

I knew, because I had seen them, that the Tibetan pilgrims carried prayer wheels that looked a little like soup cans mounted on sticks. They spun these wheels incessantly. They wore cowboy hats and porkpie hats and conical fur hats and ten-gallon hats and skimmers and bowlers and fedoras. Sometimes a pilgrim wore just a flap of cloth in, say, tartan plaid or neon pink, draped loosely over the head like a dinner napkin over a fencepost. Men and women alike wore long silky braids down their backs interwoven with brightly colored strands of cloth; they wore colorful striped skirts over their trousers, and bright vests and turquoise earrings and silver bracelets and necklaces of carnelian and agate; they wore high felt boots and sometimes cowboy boots and sometimes sneakers and once in a while they went barefoot. Sometimes they wrapped their long braids around the tops of their heads like fabulous tiaras. I saw plump bare-armed shaven-headed monks in saffron robes. I saw grannies in cotton wimples of the sort you see in seventeenth-century Dutch portraits. (Some of the grannies wore headdresses *exactly* like that of Vermeer's *Girl with a Pearl Earring*.) I saw men with Incan faces who'd poked a hole in each earlobe, fed a length of string through the hole, then hung a heavy piece of turquoise from either end of the string. They loped along the streets of Tibet, turquoise swinging.

Most of the pilgrims had traveled to Lhasa on foot, and most came from extremely far away. Nevertheless, they walked into the city with their hands clasped comfortably behind their backs as though they were just finishing up an afternoon stroll. Some of them spun their prayer wheels; some of them led little tangle-haired Lhasa apsos on rawhide leashes. Some of them came these long distances not walking but prostrating themselves the entire journey. The pilgrim stepped out the front door of his little house in a village hundreds of miles away from here, lay down on his belly, slid his hands out, and touched his forehead to the ground. Then he stood up, placed his feet where his hands had been, knelt down, and stretched himself out on his belly again. And he repeated the process over and over until he reached the city of Lhasa, creeping along the ground like a caterpillar. Some of the supplicants wore leather aprons to keep their clothes from wearing out on the roads; some wore wooden paddles strapped to their hands to protect the skin of their palms. Some particularly zealous pilgrims bound their lower legs together to prevent themselves from committing the crime of actually taking a step forward. They entered the city this way, crowding the boulevards and alleys, and when you walked through Lhasa, you had to be careful not to step on them. They circled the city a prescribed number of times (a hundred and eight, a thousand, maybe thirty-two—whatever seemed right to the individual pilgrim), prostrating themsleves along body length by body length until finally they arrived at the temple, where they would continue to prostrate themselves, sometimes for hours, kneeling, lying down, sliding their hands out in front of themselves, and standing up again with blackened palms pressed together in the position of prayer.

I knew all this because I had seen it, and what had struck me most about the Tibetan pilgrims was the look in their eyes. There is in the Tibetan gaze a vivid clarity, a gamesome look of wildness and freedom and good humor. These pilgrims had just walked possibly hundreds of miles and had been sleeping out under the stars and the birch trees for months on end, and yet somehow they didn't look fatigued or pained or put out or self-congratulating. They didn't look self-conscious in any way. They looked fresh and full of energy. Their cheeks were the color of pomegranates and had developed a kind of polished shell of hardness, like a varnish against the wind and sun. And despite the fact that they most likely had not had the benefit of a shelter or roof for ages, they looked extremely happy. When they weren't smiling, they were laughing. What they were doing was entirely natural to them and they looked delighted to be doing it, to be sliding along Lhasa's streets on their shirt buttons. For a Tibetan Buddhist, the visit to Lhasa was one of life's high points. This big city was as alien to them as it was to me, and now that they had reached it, they were every bit as fascinated by what they saw as I was. The day that I had come here by myself, I stood in front of the temple unabashedly staring.

The pilgrims had stared unabashedly too. They stood before the temple and bowed and prostrated and kowtowed over and over in a ceremony that had been going on for centuries, but as they enacted their repetitive prayerful motions in service and sacrifice to a higher enlightenment, they were looking around them in wonder, gawking at the fascinating scene, at the other pilgrims from other parts of Tibet, and at the scores of foreign tourists—Japanese, Germans, British, Americans like me—who had come here to gawk at them. Their bodies were going through the motions of prayer in pursuit of a more transcendent reality, but in their eyes, I saw a firm preoccupation with *this* reality. Their eyes were to blame. Like me, they couldn't stop *looking*.

Now, today, with a blindfold over my eyes, I stood in front of the temple and saw none of it. This was an experience of another sort. I absorbed information that I hadn't noticed before: the unceasing sibilant whisper of hundreds of pilgrims' hands sliding along the paving stones as they stretched out to lie down. I had seen the pieces of cardboard and cloth and wood that they used to protect their hands, but I hadn't registered fully the pleasing sound that all that protective matter made. It was the sound of a hundred besoms being lightly dragged along the pavement, the sound of a swan's great wings stirring the air as he passes overhead. On my first visit to the temple I hadn't really noticed the constant monotone lowing of a holy horn being blown by a monk, how soft and melancholy and *human* it sounded, like a secret, lovelorn sigh accidentally picked up by a public-address system.

I was dying to remove my blindfold and have another look around. I wanted to see the pilgrims in their wild haberdashery. I wanted to see them seeing us, the three blind visitors. Surely we would be drawing a few stares by now. But I had vowed to follow this experiment through. Knowing that there was so much activity going on around me and not being able to see any of it made me feel faceless and featureless, like a child who in covering his eyes with his hands believes he's become invisible. I asked the girls if they knew what was happening here and did they know what it looked like. They said they knew what was going on but they could only imagine what it looked like. I tried to tell them what it looked like, and as I spoke, Choden occasionally punctuated my narrative with her polite and somewhat automatic "Oh, ha," which had the effect of making me think, *Why am I telling them this?* It occurred to me that maybe they didn't give a damn what the scene looked like. Maybe they were happy with their own experience of it. But on my previous visit to the temple, I had been so captivated by the visuals of the scene that I selfishly went on describing it to them, perhaps as a way of seeing it again myself. When I finished talking, Yangchen said in her extremely polite way, "Thank you very much for telling us," and announced it was time for us to enter the temple. With their canes, the girls picked their way carefully through the crowd. "Now we are in the entrance to Jokhang Temple," Yangchen said. "The ground has changed. You feel it with feet and stick."

The toe of my shoe hit something like a step. "Is this a step?" I said. "Yah."

Hands on my wrists, the girls directed me verbally: Step up, turn here, stop, straight now, spin this prayer wheel, duck your head. Just as they knew the city by heart, they knew the temple by heart. The sounds in the temple seemed closer to our faces than the sounds outside, and each time we moved into a narrow space I could hear the low voices of pilgrims gathering in a tighter circle around us, almost like a whispering in our ears. I heard small bells jingling and a baby howling somewhere ahead of us. I heard again the sound of splashing liquid. Yangchen, who had respectfully stopped her humming as soon as we entered the temple, said, "Now we are in front of statue of Buddha." How did she know? "We smell the beer the people are giving the Buddha."

"Beer?"

Choden said, "Yah. Some Buddha, they need a beer. But not really. We just pour some beer on them in case it is true! Ha-ha." It sounded to me as though the pilgrims were hurling entire pints of beer against the Buddha's plump, laconic face. I smelled something savory cooking.

"No. That is smell of butter lamp. In the temple there's many butter lamp. Like a candle made from yak butter. You feel the floor got slippery because of the yak butter spilled?"

Sure enough, the floor was slippery under my feet. "I don't think I've ever seen a yak," I said.

"Not?"

"No, not. And if I keep this blindfold over my eyes, I never will see a yak."

"Ha, Rose," Yangchen said mirthlessly, because my joke was really not very funny. "Funny you."

A woman's voice spoke roughly and loudly close to my ear, and then she let out a high burst of laughter that sounded like a rooster saying, literally, *Cock-a-doodle-doo.* I asked the girls what the woman had said.

"She has asked us are you a blind foreigner or not a blind. We told her you are yes blind!"

The girls snickered a long time at their own bald-faced lie. I could hear two men whispering behind us. Though I couldn't see anything, I knew we had drawn a group of spectators. Someone with very rough fingers grabbed my arm and thrust a handful of warm coins into my palm. I was speechless for a moment, and then I said, "Thanks a lot," because I didn't know what else to say. As we walked on, I heard pitying tsk-tsking sounds from sighted pilgrims making their rounds of the temple. I imagined they were saying to one another, *Look at those three pathetic blindies, and one of them's a helpless old foreigner who has to be dragged about by the other two.*

I asked the girls what the people were saying about us. They hesitated; I knew they were reluctant to tell me. "Well, they have said we are blind people," Yangchen said diplomatically. "And that they will pray and we should pray."

We went up some stairs and down again. Footsteps followed us. Cymbals, or maybe it was kitchen pots and lids, crashed somewhere off to the right. To the left I heard the sound of a cowbell being vigorously hit with a stick. I heard someone wheezing just behind me, and now, instead of feeling I was in a boat moving over the water, I felt I was moving under the water. I heard a kind of squawking, more bells ringing. Other unidentifiable noises floated spookily by us. It was like passing through a particularly chaotic house of horrors. I kept expecting to be struck in the face by something very unpleasant. Suddenly Choden lifted my hand and put it down on a table scattered with cold coins.

"Rose, do you feel money?" she said. "Some people make donation here for Buddha."

Some of the coins felt sticky, probably with either beer or yak butter. "I will make a donation too," I said, dropping onto the table the coins that my blindness had moments ago attracted, and then instantly I regretted it, because what if it was bad karma to give away coins that another person had donated to you in pious pity? But if I tried to take the coins back now, it might look as though I were stealing from Buddha, and anyway, how would I be able to tell my coins from the coins that had already been there?

Choden continued holding my hand as we walked on, and soon she lifted it onto something cold and metallic. "Rose, you hold this!" It was some kind of bar. "Now you turn it around and around. This is prayer wheel."

I did as I was told, heard a soft rumbling sound as the huge metal prayer wheel turned, and then I was led up what felt like a steep pile of large rocks and down the other side. It was actually a rough staircase, like a stile.

"Up and down, up and down," Yangchen said with amusement.

I had the sense that we had entered an area that was very dark, but possibly it was simply the effect of the changing sound. Voices began to seem extremely close around us; noises became very clear. I felt as though we were walking inside a large drainpipe. I heard men's voices singing loudly in prayer, a muttering repetitive kind of droning. We turned more large prayer wheels. High-pitched bells rang out frantically. We went down more stairs, and Yangchen said in an almost incantatory way, "Down, down, down." As I walked I felt something slender and firm rub against my hand and somehow I realized that it was the bill of Choden's baseball cap.

"Did you take your cap off, Choden?"

"Yes. When we go in the temple we have to take off our cap head."

"From respect," Yangchen added.

"Yah, respect."

I heard more voices praying in unison and asked the girls what exactly they were saying. *"Om mani,"* Yangchen said, abbreviating the mantra. "Some of them been praying five and four years."

"You mean here in the temple?"

"Yah and also anywhere."

"You mean they pray for that many years without stopping?"

"No stopping."

I asked her what *om mani padme hum* actually meant.

"I cannot translate. It is something very old. People who had big sins pray this."

The people—it sounded like a group of men—were praying at a fast pace. Tom Waits seemed to be among them, growling and groaning. Yangchen joined the prayer, whispering under her breath—if she couldn't continually hum a tune while in the temple, at least she could pray, which in Tibetan sounded like just another form of humming. I could feel that the room we were in now was extremely crowded. Several times my feet knocked soundlessly against soft objects that felt like overstuffed pillows, but I soon realized that the objects were actually body parts and that all the people in this room were sitting or lying on the floor. I could hear at a level around my knees a lot of rustling and coughing and limbs shifting amid the thrumming drone of the prayers.

The girls began to lead me very carefully, Yangchen in front and Choden behind. We walked single file and linked by the hands through the crowd of people. My feet got tangled in something that felt like a plastic grocery bag, and I tripped and fell heavily forward against Yangchen, who in turn stumbled and stepped on one of the sitting people, triggering a loud snarl of protest.

"Oh! I am falling down onto one grandfather!" Yangchen muttered with distress. "My cane got crazy."

Myself, I couldn't imagine how her cane was finding any reliable pathway here at all. Choden's cane kept nipping at the backs of my ankles and scratching at my shoes and tapping the insides of my knees, and at one complicated moment, the cane goosed me completely. We bumbled along, leading one another like the Bible's accursed blind sinners.

Choden whispered just behind my left ear, "These people are praying something special. It is a special day. They have said they need some money."

"They are asking *us* for money?" I said, incredulous.

"Asking everyone."

"But we are poor blind people," I said. "We are supposed to be asking *them* for money."

This sent the girls into another unholy fit of giggles. They seemed to find it incredibly funny that I was passing myself off as blind. We staggered forward, giggling and lurching, tripping and groping at one another. There were so many people packed into this small space that the air was hot and humid and smelled of sweat and leather and yak butter. I heard tom-toms thumping at a slight distance and, again, tinkling little bells. A man's voice said something loudly and, to my ears, roughly beside us. Choden stopped in her tracks, responded to the voice, and then suddenly her voice was rising up from below my right elbow. "The man has said my shoe is not tied correctly." She had crouched down to tie the shoe.

As I stood waiting for Choden to be ready so that we could continue stumbling onward through the darkness of our blindness, I wanted to see the people in the room with us. I wanted to see their faces, and particularly their eyes. So much valuable information is reflected in a person's eyes. How could I know what was really going on here without seeing that? I could imagine it, yes, but as fabulous as imagination is, I thought, there is no substitute for sight.

Once we were outside again in the square in front of the temple I removed my blindfold and thanked the girls for the tour. Yangchen said, "Now you know how is it to be blind?"

"I have a much better idea of it, thanks to you."

They smiled. It was strange to me now to see their faces after having come to know their personalities without looking at them. They both looked much younger than they sounded. Their damaged eyes were not expressive but their mouths were extremely so; their smiles revealed pride, eagerness, expectation, and excitement. I had forgotten what they were wearing and was surprised again to see the jeans and the plaid shirts. They stood with their hands laid one upon the other on the tops of their white canes, like weary lumberjacks resting on the butts of their axes.

With my blindfold finally removed, I thought the square looked even brighter than it had the last time I was here. Lhasa is a city of short buildings situated on a flat plain. In the distance, the towering mountains are always visible, blue at their bases and capped with snow. A few misshapen clouds, like crumpled balls of paper, raced low across the impossibly blue tent of the sky. In Lhasa, the sun always seems to be directly overhead. The air is thin and dry and therefore sound carries clearly and easily. The buildings around the square were constructed of mud bricks the size of bread loaves and painted white. Everything in Lhasa looked crisp, if not entirely clean.

An elderly woman approached us and peered unabashedly at the two blind girls and at me. As the girls and I conversed, the woman's gaze jumped from my face to theirs in a baffled, figuring way. She squinted in the sunlight and shaded her eyes with her hand, the better to understand what she was seeing. Apprehension clouded her wrinkled face. Finally she asked Yangchen and Choden what language they were speaking. English, they said. The woman put her crooked fingers to her lips and stared at their blind eyes and then at me, confused and concerned. She seemed to be thinking, *They are Tibetan and blind and can speak English. I am Tibetan and not blind and I cannot speak English.* She looked distinctly as though she thought an elaborate trick was being played on her.

We headed back toward the Braille Without Borders campus, the girls still leading me by the arms. I asked them to teach me a Tibetan song, a request that delighted Yangchen. "We will teach a song that is easy and very short," she said, "because otherwise you will have to remember too much and then you are going to become annoying."

I explained to Yangchen the grammatical details of the word *annoyed*. Correcting herself, she said, "And then you are going to be annoyed," and she began singing her short and easy song. This is what I heard: *Mnachntso namaringnanatso dela zongsong. Ngala chongstiyo. Dendo zomngyo. Chongna.* When I attempted to sing all this back to her, she and Choden hooted louder and longer than they had all day. I asked them if I had sung it wrong.

"Well, not so wrong. But, okay, some small mistakes. When we have some party we sing this and we are very happy and we wish each other good things."

We practiced the song a bit and as we walked I was struck again by how cheerful and good-natured the two girls were.

We came upon a small open square where three Chinese soldiers sat playing cards beneath a tree in front of a Tibetan restaurant. China's presence was everywhere evident in Lhasa. Much of the city's infrastructure—the roads, the telecommunications—had been built by the Chinese military, and the signs on Lhasa's shop fronts now displayed more Chinese characters than Tibetan. But many of the Chinese who lived in Tibet seemed to have about them the glum, bored, slightly resentful air of the incarcerated. They looked as though they were just killing time here, waiting until they scraped together enough money to hightail it back to Beijing. The soldiers smoked cigarettes and thumbed lethargically through their fans of worn playing cards.

A woman wearing an apron appeared in the doorway of the restaurant. She was deftly peeling an apple with a ten-inch meat cleaver. When she saw the two blind girls with their white canes, her face ignited with interest. She turned and called to her coworkers inside the restaurant that a couple of blind kids were passing by. The coworkers quickly appeared in the doorway and sized up the girls literally from head to toe as we approached. They zeroed in on the girls' faces, staring at their corrupted eyes, trying to determine what exactly was the matter with them. The expressions on the workers' faces registered a complicated mix of fascination, fear, pity, disgust, and even a touch of malice. The woman in the apron stood with her hands frozen in the air, apple in one hand, cleaver in the other.

It's impossible for one human being to really know what is passing through another's mind, and so it would be unfair for me to tell you what the restaurant workers were thinking. Yet I felt strongly that, in their eyes and in their expressions, I could read what they were thinking: *If those kids can't see anything, how are they out on the street walking around like the rest of us? It must be awful being them with the world totally dark all the time and not knowing where they're going and constantly bumping into things. They'll never be able to ride a motorbike or drive a car or see the television. How would they know if I was to throw a stone at them? I could do it and they wouldn't know it was me. If I threw a stone, would they react? How can they think if they can't see the world? Can they talk? If they can hear, they must be able to talk. Maybe they can't hear either.*

The woman in the apron said something loudly to our backs as we moved off down the street. I didn't understand what she said and asked the girls to translate for me. Yangchen said, "She has said we must be sad that we are blind."

Although I was sure I knew the answer already, I asked the girls if they were indeed sad that they were blind. "No!" Choden said, her round pink cheeks glowing in the sunlight. "I am happy I am blind. I am lucky."

Why did she feel lucky?

"Because," Yangchen said, "we could come to Lhasa and learn new things with the other blind students. If we were not blind, we would still be sitting in our countries only helping at home and doing nothing. So, we are lucky."

It *was* a matter of luck for them. Sabriye and Paul had provided them with a rare opportunity for an education. Many sighted children in their villages hadn't had anywhere near the opportunities they had had. The blind students at BWB had sighted brothers and sisters, many of them illiterate, who were stuck in their mountain villages with nothing to occupy their minds but the milking of yaks. It was a complete reversal of social tradition that the blind village children were the ones suddenly being given an opportunity, but it was also precisely because they were blind that they were allowed to leave their villages. Their blindness made them undesirable. Many families wanted nothing more than to be rid of their blind children, and so in a sense the children's blindness had given them an escape route. And for the first time in Tibetan history, the blind children were beginning to understand that their blindness did not make them inferior.

We continued walking, the girls still leading me because, although I could now see, I had no idea where I was. A group of teenage boys turned their heads to stare at Yangchen and Choden and their white canes; they made some comments and then laughed loudly. I asked the girls what the boys had said. Yangchen answered calmly, "Anyway, we don't care what they say. We can read in the dark. Can they?"

At the corner where I had to turn right to go to my hotel and they had to turn left to go to the school, I took a photograph of the two girls, thanked them again for their time, and we said good-bye. I watched them for a while as they walked arm in arm away from me down the street, their white canes waving methodically before them. Choden and Yangchen were fully aware that they were being stared at everywhere they went. They knew they were being ridiculed by some, pitied by some, and despised by many. They knew they were outcasts, yet they walked cheerfully on, unfazed by the fear and the contempt of others.

# For the Benefit of
# Those Who See

In the year 1880, Phineas Taylor Barnum added a new attraction to his popular traveling circus and freak show: the Wild Men of Borneo. Dubbed Waino and Plutanor by their longtime handler, the Wild Men were two dwarf brothers, each of whom, fully grown, reached only forty inches in height and forty-five pounds in weight—approximately the size of a five-year-old child. The Wild Men were neither wild nor from Borneo; they were born on a farm in Mount Vernon, Ohio, and, as young adults, were sold by their mother to a passing showman and promoter. Their real names were Hiram and Barney Davis, born in 1825 and 1827, respectively. The brothers were widely described as being "mentally deficient," which could mean several things but which I take to mean of very low intelligence. They were an extremely odd-looking pair, judging from their photographs. They had big-boned faces, very wide, flat foreheads, short necks, receding chins, large noses, and small lopsided eyes—all facets of the warping dysmorphia of some congenital disorders. Their countenances held something of the severe, misshapen cast of the mummified faces of Seti I and Ramses II. Their skinny little bodies were chimplike, with sloping shoulders and dangling arms. Their long straight hair grew nearly to their waists. Stunted as they were, their claim to fame was that they had immense physical strength; they were said to be able to lift three hundred pounds apiece. Their extremely popular act in Barnum's freak show consisted mainly of feats of strength—wrestling fully grown men to the ground and lifting audience members over their heads. (This while dressed in horizontal-striped ballet tights and singlets.) So bizarre and fascinating were the Wild Men of Borneo that in the years they were with Barnum's circus, their act earned them a total of two hundred thousand dollars, a true fortune at the time.

In November of 1887, Annie Sullivan took her seven-year-old student, Helen Keller, on a visit to P. T. Barnum's circus. By all accounts, Keller was a pretty, impeccably dressed child with ribbons in her hair and a wreath of auburn ringlets curling about her forehead. At that time, long before her eyes had been surgically removed and replaced with painted glass orbs, the only physical sign of Keller's blindness was that her left eye protruded slightly beyond the natural seat of its socket.* Sullivan had already made great progress with Keller, helping her to transform herself from a brutish, emotionally volatile, inarticulate enigma to a charming, well-behaved little girl able to communicate intelligent thoughts and desires. In a letter to a friend, Sullivan wrote of their visit to the circus: of the riders, the clowns, the tightrope walkers they met, the many animals they saw, and of how delighted Helen was at being allowed to touch the lions, elephants, and monkeys. On being told that the lion cubs would grow up to be fierce and aggressive, Keller responded, "I will take the baby lions home and teach them to be mild," quite as her teacher had done with her.† Sullivan declared that at Barnum's circus, they had had "the time of our lives!" The excursion was a great pleasure for everyone

---

*Likely the reason that photographs of Helen Keller in her youth show the right side of her face markedly more often than they show the left.

†In her autobiography *Teacher*, Keller claimed that as a child she was so uncontrollable that she had "acted like a demon" and knocked out two of Annie Sullivan's teeth.

involved. Except, it seems, for one of the Wild Men of Borneo. According to Sullivan, upon meeting Helen Keller, "the Wild Man of Borneo shrank from her sweet little face in terror."

Blindness, more than any other physical handicap, has been terrifying even the most intelligent and enlightened people since the beginning of time. The common negative reaction that the sighted have toward the blind is visceral, and the social status of millions of blind people has been decided more by sighted people's emotional misprision of them than by any qualities or inabilities inherent in the blind person. The response we have to the blind is reflexive and prepotent. It is a hysterical projection that continually clouds our reason.

In her intelligent and vastly informative history *The Imprisoned Guest: Samuel Howe and Laura Bridgman, the Original Deaf-Blind Girl*, published in 2001, Elisabeth Gitter described the self-referential quality of unease that sighted people often feel around the blind:

> Because the blind cannot participate in the social code of affiliative facial signals, in the ritual exchange of nods, smiles, and glances, they deprive the sighted of the sense of a seen—and therefore secure— self. Not finding themselves mirrored in the eyes and expressions of the blind, the sighted may experience a sense of dread mixed with guilty anger and revulsion, a feeling of uncanniness.

On the ramifications of this unease, Pierre Villey, a blind French professor of literature at the University of Caen, wrote in *The World of the Blind* in 1930,

> The sighted person judges the blind not for what they are but by the fear blindness inspires.... Stronger than all external observations, the revolt of his sensibility in the face of "the most atrocious of maladies" fills a sighted person with prejudice and gives rise to a thousand leg-

ends. The sighted person imagines himself struck by blindness....An abyss opens up before him.

Passed down over eons, the prejudice against the blind is, like all clichés, difficult to bury.

Traditionally, the blind have been perceived and portrayed in one of three stereotypic ways: as mystical soothsayers endowed with supernatural and thus potentially dangerous powers; as helpless ineducable idiots fit only for pity and mockery; or as vagrant beggars with base morals and uncanny gifts for cunning and deception. These portraits, which sometimes overlap, are confusing and even contradictory. As the blind author Georgina Kleege observed, "The blind are either supernatural or subhuman, alien or animal."

Since the beginning of recorded history, the blind simply have not come off very well. I'll start with the Old Testament,[*] which gives a rather bleak picture of their situation. The exclusion of the blind, along with every other unworthy cripple, from the altar of God is decreed right up front in Leviticus:

> For no one who has a blemish shall draw near, a man blind or lame, or one who has a mutilated face or a limb too long, or a man who has an injured foot or an injured hand, or a hunchback, or a dwarf, or a man with a defect in his sight [in case "a man blind" wasn't clear enough] or an itching disease or scabs or crushed testicles...He may eat the bread of his God, both of the most holy and of the holy things, but he shall not come near the veil or approach the altar because he has a blemish, that he may not profane my sanctuaries.

---

[*]I could, I think, start with almost any ancient text—*The Epic of Gilgamesh, The Tale of Genji, The Pyramid Texts,* or *The Avestan Gathas*—and effectively make the same point.

The Lord considered the blind tainted, but King David outright despised them and wanted them all ostracized or, better yet, dead:

> David took the stronghold of Zion, that is, the city of David. And David said on that day, "Whoever would smite the Jeb'usites, let him get up the water shaft to attack the lame and the blind, who are hated by David's soul." Therefore it is said, "The blind and the lame shall not come into the house."

Blindness was considered not only a mark of opprobrium but a most fitting punishment for disobedience to God.

In the book of Genesis when the two angels disguised as earthly men go to the city of Sodom to pass judgment on its wayward people, Lot invites them to spend the night in his house. Before the night is over, a crowd of men, with the malign intent intrinsic to Sodomites, gathers outside Lot's house and demand to see the two visitors. Lot refuses to produce them. Enraged, the crowd threatens him, but before the men can get their hands on him, the two angels come to the rescue and strike "with blindness the men who were at the door of the house, both small and great, so that they wearied themselves groping for the door." The angels could as easily have incapacitated the men by paralyzing them from the necks down or casting them all into epileptic fits of extended duration. But no, blindness was the weapon of choice against bad character; it delivered a uniquely insulting sting.

In the New Testament, in the Gospel according to Mark, Jesus restored sight to a blind man. Upon meeting the man, the disciples' first question had been, "Master, who did sin, this man, or his parents, that he was born blind?" The question was only natural, because what *other* possible reason for congenital blindness could there be? In biblical times, the moral implication of blindness was explicit: It was God's punishment for guilt, sin, and transgression.

I scoured the Old and New Testaments both on the off chance that there might be something positive in them about the blind. I found a few miraculous healings and a few monitory temporary blindings, such as that of Paul, whose sight was quickly restored to him when he reversed his position and professed his faith in the Lord. These, however, are not positive attitudes toward the blind—they are only positive attitudes toward sight. I did find a few charitable gestures toward the blind: "Thou shalt not curse the deaf nor put a stumbling block before the blind" and "I was eyes to the blind, and feet was I to the lame." But these are not positive either, unless pity and paternalism are positive.

In Greek and Roman mythology, in which a staggering amount of eye-gouging takes place, the report on the blind improves just a little. Still, in a great many cases, blindness is the fate of anyone who manifests an egregious fault or character flaw, or it is meted out as punishment for a crime or personal offense against the gods. With a sharpened stick, Odysseus gouges out the one large eye of the giant Cyclops Polyphemus to punish him for having eaten five or six of Odysseus's devoted men as well as for sorely violating the strict rules of Achaean hospitality: Wiping his enormous mouth on his sleeve, idly picking human bones from between his tombstone-size teeth, the boorish Cyclops had mockingly told Odysseus that as his "guest-gift," he would finish the meal off by eating Odysseus too.

Polymestor, the king of Thrace, is also guilty of rough hospitality. Temporarily entrusted with the care and safety of King Priam's young son Polydorus and the gold and other precious treasures the boy brings with him, Polymestor flings the child off a cliff and into the sea, thereby ensuring that all that treasure will be his. When Polydorus's mother, Hecuba, gets wind of the murder, she orders the women of Troy to kill Polymestor's children, and then, for good measure, she gouges his eyes out with her own hands, saying, "His debt is paid, and I have revenge."

Witnessing a goddess in the nude was a common cause of human blindness in Greek mythology. When Erymanthos, the son of Apollo, sees Aphrodite bathing, she blinds him for the outrage. When Tiresias stumbles upon Athena bathing, he pays the same penalty.* Tiresias's mother begs Athena to unblind her son; Athena declares that she is unable to do so, but, as feeble compensation, she cleans Tiresias's ears, which gives him the ability to understand birdsong and, by extension, the gift of prophecy—so often a power associated with the blind. (Homer's purported blindness was believed to have brought him a kind of sixth sense, a connection to the world of the gods, and hence his poetic gift, his insight, and his wisdom.)

To ancient minds, blindness was a greater punishment than death, an ongoing mark of shame, an enduring torture, the lowest state to which a person could possibly sink, a depth from which there was no return. Realizing all the terrible deeds he has unwittingly committed, Oedipus does the only proper thing: He tears out his own eyes, crying, "Too long you looked on the ones you never should have seen, blind to the ones you longed to see, to know! Blind from this hour on! Blind in the darkness—blind!" Oedipus carried on that way for the rest of his life, never quite adapting to it, endlessly horrified and surprised to find that he was blind. Putting a fine point on just how profane, insulting, and significant a revenge the act of blinding was, Alcmene made the extra effort to gouge out the eyes of Eurystheus, her son Hercules's nemesis, even *after* his head had been severed from his body.

The ancient Greek word for blindness is *átē,* but in Homer and in the mythology of later authors, the word suggests metaphorical rather

---

*This is one of several explanations for the cause of Tiresias's blindness; others include his failure to take Hera's side in a disagreement between Hera and Zeus about sexual pleasure, and the general annoyance of the gods when he revealed their secrets.

than physical blindness, a confusion of the mind rather than a failing of the eyes. *Átē* has no exact translation, but its chief meanings are "folly," "delusion," "mental ignorance," "passion," "disaster," "ruin," and "calamity."* All in all, *átē* is a dark, mysterious state. The historian Moshe Barasch addressed the significance of *átē* in the early formation of the reputation of the blind. Most important is "the belief that both blindness and madness, being either god-sent or the outcome of the intervention of demons, have something of a numinous, supernatural character."

Prejudices and preconceptions inevitably evolve over time, but across the ages, society's attitude toward blindness has remained hostile. The idea that blindness is punishment for a sin or a crime, a mark of mysticism, or evidence of idiocy persisted into the medieval period and well beyond.

The World Health Organization estimates that 285 million people in the world are visually impaired: 246 million of them have what's known as low vision, and 39 million are completely blind. It should come as no surprise that 90 percent of the world's blind or visually impaired people live in developing countries. Ethiopia has the world's highest rate of blindness. India has 18.7 million blind citizens. Nearly 51 percent of the world's blindness is caused by cataracts, one of the most easily curable ocular disorders. To put the present status of the world's blind in perspective, nine out of ten blind or visually impaired children in developing countries have no access whatever to education. *Because* they are blind. The United States has the lowest rate of blindness in the world, and yet among Americans, blindness is the most feared physical affliction, following only AIDS and cancer. (There is, I suspect, a direct correlation here; the less familiar we are with a thing, the more frightening it becomes.)

---

*Richard E. Doyle, *Átē, Its Use and Meaning: A Study in the Greek Poetic Tradition from Homer to Euripides* (New York: Fordham University Press, 1984).

When I learned, early in my research for this book, that the world's first school for the blind was founded in 1785, I was surprised. Because we have known for millennia that education is one of the fundamental requirements for the development of humanity, 1785 struck me as woefully late in the greater scheme of human history. What didn't surprise me was that this first school was founded in Paris, for when it comes to the blind, the French were perhaps the most progressive people in Europe, if not the world.

In her fiercely well-researched study *The Blind in French Society from the Middle Ages to the Century of Louis Braille,* Zina Weygand gives a minutely detailed view of the social perception of the blind in France in the second half of the second millennium. Motivated by the question "Why is it that today, in a 'disenchanted' world, blind people still face irrational behavior that partially determines their place in our society?," Weygand, a scholar of seemingly limitless patience and determination, apparently unearthed and analyzed every extant receipt, ledger, government certificate, theater script, novel, private letter, ticket stub, tax roll, invoice, treatise, religious text, scholarly text, petition, and picture pertaining to the blind in France over a five-hundred-year period.

Beginning in the thirteenth century, the blind became the focus of what Weygand calls "profane theater" in France, the farcical and often vulgar entertainment for the general public. In these comedies the blind man was always a beggar, buffoonish, drunken, vice-ridden, outwardly pathetic, and yet full of wile and deceit, playing disingenuously on the emotions of passersby. The belief that blindness was a punishment for sin was still strong at this time. "It is therefore not surprising," Weygand writes, "that medieval literature was able to cast the blind beggar—whose disability symbolized blindness of the spirit and the dimming of intelligence—as a negative character who could be mercilessly laughed at by the public of farces and fabliaux."

That the blind were considered fair targets for ridicule and contempt is beautifully illustrated in a scene from *Journal d'un bourgeois de Paris,* known in English as *A Parisian Journal.* The anonymous author recorded a street event (he called it "an entertainment") on the rue Saint-Honoré in the year 1425. Four blind men were given batons, were placed in a pen with a piglet, and were told that if they could kill the piglet, they could keep it.

> And this made for a battle so strange...because however much they thought to strike the piglet, they struck each other, and if they had really been armed, they'd have killed each other. On Saturday, following the Sunday vigils, the said blind men were led through Paris in suits of armor and were preceded by a large banner on which there was the image of a pig, and in front of them, a man playing a tabret.

At the same time that the blind were being mocked and taunted, charitable public institutions such as hospices and hospitals were being founded all over France at the behest of the Catholic Church, and as part of this trend, the first organizations specifically for the aid of the blind were established. In the mid-thirteenth century, the just, crusading, and pathologically pious* king Louis IX lobbied for the foundation of a hospice that would house, feed, and generally support three hundred blind Parisians. Because of the number of inmates, the hospice came to be called the Hôpital des Quinze-Vingts. In exchange for their protection and care, the blind inmates of the Quinze-Vingts were re-

---

*How else to describe a man who was moved to purchase from the emperor of Constantinople all the existing accoutrements of Christ's crucifixion: the crown of thorns, parts of the true cross, the holy lance, and the holy sponge? How else to describe a king who was said to have attended mass twice daily, loved sermons, surrounded himself at all times with chanting priests (even when traveling), fed the poor and the sick with his own hands, and had a habit of passing out hair shirts to his friends?

quired to pray concertedly for their benefactors and to venture into the city seeking alms and further donations. On these trips into the city, the Quinze-Vingts blind wore special uniforms identifying them as legitimate and respectable inmates of the hospice, as opposed to those shiftless bands of blind beggars who for centuries had been plaguing the streets of Paris with their pitiable cries and their battered tin cups. The Quinze-Vingts blind would prevail upon passersby with the relatively inoffensive plea "For the Quinze-Vingts, the bread of God!" Their religious slant and their favor with the crown brought them success enough that other organizations for the blind began to copy their model and compete with them for funds and donations. Weygand argues that although the establishment of the Quinze-Vingts was the first move the French monarchy ever made in aid of the handicapped, the hospice's focus on alms-collecting further cemented the already strong association between blindness and begging. "Even privileged, the blind of the Quinze-Vingts remained beggars, and as such, they were still objects of mockery as much as pity."

Medieval literature is rife with blind beggars. Dante's vivid description of them in *Purgatorio* is surely an accurate representation of the methods and demeanor of the average European blind beggar at the beginning of the fourteenth century:

Covered with sackcloth vile they seemed to me,
And one sustained the other with his shoulder,
And all of them were by the bank sustained.
Thus do the blind, in want of livelihood,
Stand at the doors of churches asking alms,
And one upon another leans his head,
So that in others pity soon may rise,
Not only at the accent of their words,
But at their aspect, which no less implores.

This "want of livelihood" persisted for at least another hundred years and into the sixteenth century before the rise of humanism and its move to eradicate poverty gave birth to the idea that the blind could—and should—work and be educated. In 1526 the Spanish humanist Juan Luis Vives published *On Assistance to the Poor,* in which this novel idea was formally articulated for the first time:

> Not even the blind shall be allowed to remain idle; there are many things they can do. Some have a literary disposition, provided that someone read to them. Let them study, for we observe that a number of them make progress in erudition that is not to be disdained. Others have a talent for music: let them sing and play string and wind instruments. Let others work at the press houses to help maneuver the wine presses, and may others do their best at the bellows in the workshops of blacksmiths. We know that the blind make boxes, baskets, trays, and cages, and that blind women spin and wind skeins. In sum, if they neither wish to be unemployed nor to flee work, they will easily find something to keep themselves occupied. Laziness or indolence, and not a bodily defect, is the only excuse they may put forward for doing nothing.

According to Weygand, Vives had no particular interest in the blind but was simply arguing that elements of society that had heretofore been deemed unemployable could in fact be economically productive. His treatise was a step toward treating the blind the same way as everyone else in society.

One of the greatest changes in the perception of the blind over the past thousand years came as a by-product of the Enlightenment's focus on reason, science, and the nature of human knowledge. Descartes and other philosophers of the age believed that human ideas were innate, imbued in them by God in the process of creation. John Locke dismissed this notion as superstition and argued instead that the principles of human knowledge were not innate but learned through both experience and the development of the five senses. The chief purpose of Locke's 1690 essay *Concerning Human Understanding* was to explore the question of the true source of human thought and ideas. In a letter responding to Locke's empiricist essay, the Irish philosopher William Molyneux posed a hypothetical question, asking Locke whether he thought that a person born blind who had learned to distinguish a cube from a sphere simply by touching them could, upon regaining his sight, distinguish the two simply by looking at them. Molyneux postulated that the answer was no. Locke agreed, and the question became the focal point of a decades-long philosophical debate concerning the origin and process of human knowledge and the role that the five senses play in human understanding. Sixteen years later another Irish philosopher, George Berkeley, joined Locke and Molyneux's consensus in his *Essay Towards a New Theory of Vision.*

> From what hath been premised it is a manifest consequence that a man born blind, being made to see, would, at first, have no idea of distance by sight; the sun and stars, the remotest objects as well as the nearer, would all seem to be in his eye, or rather in his mind.... For our judging objects provided by sight to be at any distance, or without the mind, is entirely the effect of experience, which one in those circumstances could not yet have attained to.

Molyneux, Locke, and Berkeley were all correct in their supposition that sight lost early in life cannot be effectively regained, but their arguments were not supported by any empirical evidence until 1728, when the English surgeon William Cheselden performed the modern world's first successful surgery to restore sight to a blind person. The patient was a thirteen-year-old boy born blind. When his cataracts were removed, the boy could indeed see, but as Cheselden observed,

> When he first saw, he was so far from making any judgment of distances, that he thought all objects whatever touched his eyes... as what he felt did his skin [i.e., he believed that whatever he saw was literally touching his eyes, in the same way that whatever he felt was touching his skin]... He knew not the shape of anything, nor any one thing from another, however different in shape or magnitude; but upon being told what things were, whose form he knew before from feeling, he would carefully observe, that he might know them again.

The Enlightenment inquiry into the role of the senses in the formation of human thought was scientific, theoretical, and philosophical in nature and was not inspired by any particular concern for the blind or by any attempts to improve their lives. It was, however, this debate over Molyneux's question that prompted a closer understanding of the daily experience of the blind and that eventually led to Diderot's *Letter on the Blind for the Benefit of Those Who See,* a fascinating treatise that contains probably the first formal investigation of and appreciation for a blind person as an intelligent, capable human being.

Denis Diderot, who was born in 1713, was thirty-six years old when he published *Letter on the Blind.* He was a rationalist who openly questioned the tenets, dogmas, and authority of the Church, especially its definition of the nature of God. He was a Catholic who was capable of writing "I maintain that superstition is more of an insult to God than atheism."

Much of Diderot's *Letter on the Blind* describes a visit he and a friend made to a man in Puiseaux, France, who was born blind. Upon interviewing the man and finding him intelligent and articulate, Diderot was exactly as surprised and amazed as I was two hundred and sixty years later upon meeting Sabriye Tenberken (which only confirms, I think, how ossified and entrenched society's judgments and perceptions are on this subject and how little they have changed with the passage of time). Throughout the *Letter,* the blind man goes unnamed, but many details of his life are given. The son of a professor of philosophy at the University of Paris, the blind man was "possessed of good solid sense," was married, and had a young son whom he was teaching to read with the aid of raised letters. He had many acquaintances, understood some chemistry, made his living distilling liqueurs that he sold in Paris, and attended lectures on botany at the Jardin du Roi. He was in the habit of sleeping most of the day, getting up in the late afternoon, and working most of the night. He was particular about tidiness and order in his home, and at night, after his family went to bed, he would put everything in the house in its proper place. "The difficulty the blind have in finding things that are mislaid makes them orderly," Diderot wrote. The blind man could (like many blind people) thread needles well and sew, and he had (like many blind people) a "surprising" memory for sounds and voices. According to Diderot, he was able to "distinguish as many differences in voices as we can in faces." He had an uncanny ability to determine the precise weight of an object simply by holding it in his hand and could similarly determine how much liquid a vessel could hold just by feeling it. He could operate a lathe, could dismantle and reassemble small machines, could play an unfamiliar tune merely by being told the notes, and (like many blind people) he considered himself in some respects superior to sighted people. "This blind man," Diderot wrote, "values himself as much as, and perhaps more than, we who see." On being asked whether he wouldn't like to have vision, the blind man responded (as congenitally blind people often do):

> If it were not for curiosity, I would just as soon have long arms: it seems to me my hands would tell me more of what goes on in the

moon than your eyes or your telescopes; and besides, eyes cease to see sooner than hands to touch. I would be as well off if I perfected the organ I possess, as if I obtained the organ which I am deprived of.*

Diderot was impressed by the simplicity and accuracy of the blind man's answer when asked to define what eyes actually are: "An organ on which the air has the effect that this stick has on my hand. When I place my hand between your eyes and an object, my hand is present to you, but the object is absent. The same thing happens when I reach for one thing with my stick and come across another." Diderot was also struck by how keen the man's audio perception was, how accurately he could tell where a sound was coming from, and with obvious admiration, he recounted a story about a heated argument the blind man had with his brother as a youth, during which he hurled a weighty object in the direction of the brother's voice: He hit the brother square on the forehead and knocked him out. Diderot was also astonished, as I was with Sabriye, Choden, and Yangchen, that "he is so sensitive to the least atmospheric change that he can distinguish between a street and a closed alley." Like Sabriye, the blind man of Puiseaux judged a person's appeal by his pronunciation and "charm of voice."

Eventually, displaying the inevitable impatience that blind people will if questioned too simplistically for too long about their blindness, the blind man asked Diderot and his friend a question of his own. "I perceive, gentlemen, that you are not blind. You are astonished at what I do, and why not as much at my speaking?"

Diderot did in fact wonder how the blind could speak as well as the sighted, for there is so much in language that refers to phenomena per-

---

*Helen Keller, for her part, wrote, "I am sure that if a fairy bade me choose between the sense of sight and that of touch, I would not part with the warm, endearing contact of human hands or the wealth of form, the mobility and fullness that press into my palms."

ceptible only to the eyes—the mischievous glance, for example; the wry smile; the angry frown. How can a blind person know what these are or tell one from the other? Helen Keller addressed this question at length in *The World I Live In*. On reading one of her essays, Keller's proofreader queried her use of the word *see* in the following sentence: "When I was a little girl I was taken to see a woman who was blind and paralyzed." Keller protested, "If I had said 'visit,' he would have asked no questions, yet what does 'visit' mean but 'see' *visitare?*" Defending herself for using "as much of the English language as I have succeeded in learning," Keller wrote critically of a newspaper article that announced the publication of a new magazine for the blind. The article explained that many poems and stories had to be omitted from the magazine "because they deal with sight. Allusion to moonbeams, rainbows, starlight, clouds, and beautiful scenery may not be printed, because they serve to emphasize the blind man's sense of his affliction." Keller scoffed that this was like suggesting "I may not talk about beautiful mansions because I am poor. I may not read about Paris and the West Indies because I cannot visit them in their territorial reality. I may not dream of heaven because it is possible that I may never go there. Yet a venturesome spirit impels me to use words of sight and sound whose meaning I can guess only from analogy and fancy."*

In the second section of his *Letter on the Blind*, Diderot examined

---

*More technically, Keller wrote, "The blind child—the deaf blind child—has inherited the mind of seeing and hearing ancestors—a mind measured to five senses. Therefore he must be influenced, even if it be unknown to himself, by the light, color, song which have been transmitted through the language he is taught, for the chambers of the mind are ready to receive that language.... Since the mind of the sightless is essentially the same as that of the seeing... it must supply some sort of equivalent for missing physical sensations.... Because I can understand the word 'reflect' figuratively, a mirror has never perplexed me." (The blind man of Puiseaux also seemed to understand the general concept of the mirror.) On this topic, by the way, Schopenhauer believed that an intelligent blind person could create a theory and understanding of color simply from hearing accurate descriptive statements.

the life of the British mathematician Nicholas Saunderson, who was born in 1682 and lost his sight to smallpox at the age of twelve months. Saunderson eventually became Lucasian Chair of Mathematics at Cambridge University and was widely recognized as a mathematical genius and a brilliant teacher. He was expert in Greek, Latin, and French, and wrote *The Elements of Algebra,* in which, according to Diderot, the "only signs of his blindness are the peculiarity of certain demonstrations which a sighted man would probably not have thought of." (This is surely a compliment.) He also devised an ingenious tablet for working out his mathematical calculations and algebraic formulations, which he performed with "astonishing rapidity." Saunderson lectured on Newtonian philosophy, optics, the nature of light and color, hydrostatics, astronomy, mechanics, and the theory of vision, and he wrote about the properties of lenses and the phenomenon of the rainbow. "He taught his pupils as if they could not see," Diderot wrote, "and a blind man who makes clear to the blind must be doubly lucid to the sighted." Saunderson could tell a genuine coin from a counterfeit coin simply by feeling both, even though one particular counterfeit was well enough made to have duped a sighted expert numismatist. (From this Diderot concluded that the sense of touch, "when trained, could become more delicate than sight."\*) Saunderson was able to tell the size of a space he was standing in just by its atmosphere, and he could immediately recognize a place he had stood in just once before by the sound that the walls and pavement "reflected." The entry on Saunderson in the *Biographia Britannica* of 1766 stated that he was "supposed not to entertain any great notion of revealed religion," meaning that he preferred reason and ordinary

---

\*He wrote, further, "I found that of the senses, the eye is the most superficial, the ear the most arrogant, smell the most voluptuous, taste the most superstitious and fickle, touch the most profound and the most philosophical."

experiences to scripture and religious experiences, ultimately implying he was an atheist. The *Bio Britannica* also prissily opined that while Saunderson was a vivacious and witty conversationalist, he "uttered his sentiments of men not only freely but licentiously, with a kind of contempt and disregard for decency and commonsense; and which is worse, he indulged himself in women, wine, and profane swearing to shocking excess; by which means he did more hurt to the reputation of mathematics than he did good by his eminent skill in the science." (Can the reputation of mathematics, or any other science, be damaged by a nonconforming practitioner? This seems to *me* disregard for common sense. Isaac Newton, who had also occupied the Lucasian Chair at Cambridge, was psychologically unstable, vindictive, violent of temper, depressive, and a moneylender. If I had had such complex math teachers, perhaps mathematics would have become comprehensible to me instead of remaining an occult mystery.)

Diderot never met Saunderson, who died ten years before the *Letter on the Blind* was written, but in order to explore several metaphysical questions, among them deism and the weakness of the teleological argument of design, he presumed to devise in the *Letter* a fictional dialogue between the dying Saunderson and his friend Gervaise Holmes. When Holmes speaks of the wonders of nature as evidence enough that God exists, Saunderson responds skeptically from his deathbed, "Ah, sir, don't talk to me of this magnificent spectacle, which it has never been my lot to enjoy.... If you want to make me believe in God, you must make me touch him." Anticipating Darwin by a hundred years, Diderot had Saunderson speak compellingly, and transgressively, of a theory of natural selection, the extinction of imperfect creatures, and the survival and evolution of only those creatures most fit. Creation was a random act; God did not exist.

In July of 1749, as a result of the publication of Diderot's *Letter on the Blind,* two police officers arrived at Diderot's home and searched it for manuscripts "contrary to Religion, the State, or Morals." They arrested and imprisoned him at the Château de Vincennes for three months.[*]

Though Diderot's *Letter on the Blind* was essentially a response to Molyneux's philosophical question about the perceptions of the newly sighted, it had long-ranging consequences for the blind. For the first time, a blind man had been given the opportunity to speak of his experience and to assert that his experience held its own primacy. "People try to give those born blind the gift of sight," Diderot wrote, "but, rightly considered, science would be equally advanced by questioning a sensible blind man." Oliver Sacks interpreted Diderot's *Letter* as an exercise in cultural relativism that suggested that the blind "may in their own way construct a complete and sufficient world, have a complete 'blind identity' and no sense of disability or inadequacy, and that the 'problem' of their blindness and the desire to cure this, therefore, is ours, not theirs."

---

[*]In her introduction to the 1911 edition of *Diderot's Early Philosophical Works,* the translator Margaret Jourdain offered the reader some curious and inapposite bits of information about the philosopher. It is known to anyone who has read it that the *Letter on the Blind* was formally addressed to one Madame Madeleine de Puisieux (nothing to do with the blind man of Puiseaux), who happened to be Diderot's mistress. Madame de Puisieux was a writer (Jourdain dismissed her as a "fifth-rate female scribbler") and in constant need of money; indeed, according to Jourdain, much of the writing Diderot did at that time he took on "to fill the purse of Madame de Puisieux." While Diderot was in prison, Madame de Puisieux came to visit him, and when he saw that she was dressed in her best clothing, he became suspicious. He asked her where she was going in her finery; she responded, "To a fete at Champigny." When he asked whether she was going alone, she answered, "Yes." As soon as she left him, Diderot escaped over the prison wall and found at Champigny exactly what he had feared he would: Madame de Puisieux with another lover. This story ends with Diderot climbing back over the wall into the prison. While in prison, Diderot had neither pen nor ink to write with, so he broke a slate off the wall of his prison room, ground it to powder, and mixed it with wine in a broken glass, thereby making ink. For a pen he used a toothpick he found in his pocket. And what did he do for paper? He just happened to have with him a copy of Milton's *Paradise Lost* and in its margins and blank pages he wrote his thoughts and notes. (That a man imprisoned for writing an essay on the blind should happen to have with him in his cell the work of a blind author either makes perfect sense or is so tidily coincidental and symbolic that the entire story is complete rubbish.)

The widely held assumption that blindness holds nothing but loss is quickly corrected by the testimony of the blind themselves.

Valentin Haüy, born in Paris in 1745, was a professional translator, linguist, teacher, handwriting expert, and certified interpreter of Italian, Spanish, Portuguese, German, English, Dutch, and Swedish. Fascinated by language in general, he was also versed in Latin, Greek, and Hebrew. Having taken an interest in the methods of sign language that the Abbé Charles-Michel de l'Épée devised in the 1760s to instruct his deaf-mute students, Haüy began to envision similar methods for teaching the blind. At that time, quite a few blind people of the upper classes had had the privilege of private tutors and readers, and their educational successes were well documented. Struck by Diderot's *Letter on the Blind,* Haüy hoped to make education available to blind people of all classes. As inspiration for his efforts, he cited both the blind man of Puiseaux, who had instructed his own son with raised letters, and Nicholas Saunderson, who had taught mathematics "in the midst of a circle of sighted people." In his *Essay on the Education of Blind Children,* Haüy stated that his ultimate purpose in giving the blind an education was to put "the means of subsistence in their power."*

Haüy's ultimate inspiration came in the form of a spectacle he witnessed at the St. Ovid's Fair in September 1771, in which inmates of the Quinze-Vingts hospital performed a farcical "concert" for the entertainment of fairgoers. The event was described in the *Fairground Almanac* of 1773:

---

*On the value of educating the blind in music, he wrote: "It is only the want of instruction...which reduces some of them to the necessity of wandering in the streets, from door to door, grating the ear by the aid of an ill-tuned instrument, or a hoarse voice, that they may extort an inconsiderable piece of money, which is frequently given them with an injunction to be silent."

The orchestra consisted of eight men dressed in long gowns and hold-ing pointed bonnets. A ninth was suspended in the air on a peacock and beat time (but was out of beat). Like his comrades, he had a red gown, clogs on his feet, and a big dunce cap with ass's ears. In turn, they sang amusing couplets, accompanying themselves ridiculously on the violin....In front of each blind person was a sheet of music and a lit candle. The throngs of people who came to see this farce were sometimes so large that it was necessary to place fusiliers at the coffeehouse door.

The cacophonous show left the spectators in absolute stitches. Haüy, however, was unamused. He described the event as a "public dishonor to the human race" and claimed that upon witnessing it, he vowed to "replace this ridiculous fable with truth. I will make the blind read."

Twelve years passed before Haüy, who had limited means, was pre-pared to appeal to the relatively new Philanthropic Society of Paris for assistance in founding his Royal Institution for the Young Blind. By that time, he had succeeded in teaching an intelligent seventeen-year-old blind beggar named François Le Sueur to read, write, do mathematical calculations, identify the various continents and coun-tries on specially created tactile maps, write music, and print books for other blind people. (Haüy had hired experts to help him create raised type that could be interpreted and manipulated by the blind and to develop methods of embossing raised type on wet paper.) In 1784 Haüy and Le Sueur publicly demonstrated all that Le Sueur had learned: Le Sueur read aloud from a book of type printed in relief, wrote down dictated sentences, and performed mathematical calculations on a device that Haüy had perfected. His demonstration impressed his audience, and, with the support of the Philanthropic Society of Paris, Haüy's group of students grew. Le Sueur was hired as their teacher, and Haüy's free school for "those born blind" officially opened in 1785. The school accepted blind students from all the social classes and instructed them all in the same manner with no distinction or favoritism. In addition to academics, the students learned crafts such as string-making, net-making, knitting, printing, and bookbinding.

In its early years, the institution weathered many upheavals (not least the French Revolution), financial setbacks, rivalries, and, once nationalized, a great deal of state interference, including the school's disastrous merging with the Hôpital des Quinze-Vingts. Control of the institution's administration was wrested from Haüy, and his students were turned into little more than sweatshop workers churning out textiles and forced to live under strict surveillance in appalling conditions. Without Haüy's authority and protection, the students suffered the same disregard the blind had always been subjected to. "These... poor wretches seemed infinitely less well taken care of than the orphans of La Pietie," wrote the German author August von Kotzebue of his visit to the institute. "The residence is big but dirty." For political reasons, Haüy was eventually completely deposed and forced to leave the school.

The machinations of the various parties vying for control of the institution, its students, and its funding were complex; as a result, the school was in turmoil for years. Suffice it to say that not until 1821 did the school return to the educational model that Haüy had envisioned. The blind were still feared, reviled, and reduced to beggary (although by 1808 begging was forbidden by law in Paris), but for once they did have a school that catered to their particular needs.

In 1819 a ten-year-old blind boy named Louis Braille entered Haüy's institution, which was now called the National Institute for Blind Youth. When he was three years old, Braille accidentally injured one of his eyes with a knife he found in his father's workshop; the eye became infected, the infection spread to his other eye, and he was left completely blind. Braille was extremely intelligent, a prize-winning student, and he was particularly gifted in the sciences. He could play the piano and the violin well. At twelve years of age, he examined a new form of tactile writing that had just been introduced to the institute. It had been developed by Nicolas Barbier de La Serre, an army officer who was searching for methods of speed writing that would be of benefit to the military; the system was based on punctiform symbols that he called night writing. Braille immediately identified the flaws of Barbier de La Serre's method, and after long experimentation he came up with a vastly improved version. Braille was said to be extremely humble and modest. In the foreword to his 1829 *Method of Writing Words, Music, and Plainsong by Means of Dots, for Use by the Blind and Arranged for Them*, Braille, who was now twenty years old and must have known that his system far surpassed Barbier de La Serre's, graciously wrote, "At the end of this work can be found a sort of stenographic system for which twelve signs suffice to write all the words in the French language. Three of these signs take up as much space as one of Mr. Barbier's. If we have signaled the advantages of our method over this inventor's, we must also say, to his credit, that it is his system that gave us the first idea for our own." Not long after Braille completed his work with the dotted alphabet and began teaching it to other students at the school, he was called for the draft by the French army. Census records state that Braille was exempted from military service because he was blind and therefore "unable to read and write."

While the blind students at the institute took quickly to the Braille method of writing (in 1837 they published the first Braille book in the world: a history of France in three volumes), it was slow to catch on with school authorities. The assistant director of the school, P. Armand Dufau, was dead set against the Braille system, claiming that it made the blind "too dependent"; he preferred instead a system invented by the Scotsman John Alston. To ensure that Alston's system and not Braille's would be adopted, Dufau burned the school's entire library—all of Haüy's raised-type books as well as all the Braille books he found. In the hope of putting a final end to the Braille system, he confiscated all of the school's Braille writing equipment.

The students at the school, most of whom had thrived on the Braille system, were horrified by Dufau's actions and staged a sort of passive protest by continuing to write notes to one another in Braille with whatever implements they could find: forks, nails, knitting needles—any pointed objects that were handy. As their punishment for writing in Braille, the students were slapped and starved, but this did not deter them. Passionate about communicating their ideas and feelings with Braille's system, they passed the method on to new students.

Joseph Gaudet, Dufau's assistant, understood the power of Braille and warned Dufau that his position might be at risk if government officials found out that the students were unanimously defying him. In addition, he pointed out, if the school could claim that one of its students had invented this new popular method of tactile writing, it would only benefit the school and boost the reputation of its administrators. Dufau saw the logic in this and altered his position: Braille was once again adopted as the primary means of communication and tutelage at the school.

Some months later, during a public lecture, Dufau praised Louis Braille's system and asked the blind students to demonstrate its effectiveness. A blind child took dictation in Braille, and then another blind child (who had not been in the room to hear the dictation) read it back. The audience was captivated but skeptical. One man called out that the whole thing was a trick and a put-on, that the children must have memorized the passage beforehand! Dufau responded by asking the doubter to produce any written material he could find in his pocket and read it out loud to the students. He did so; one blind girl wrote the text down in Braille, and another read it back exactly, word for word, "before the man even returned to his seat." It is said that the audience members were so astonished they applauded for six minutes.

The Braille method encountered a great deal of resistance internationally, and always for the same reason: It appeared to the sighted nothing at all like the print they were familiar with, and this made it somehow unacceptable. A full fifty years passed before the Universal Congress for the Improvement of the Lot of the Blind and Deaf-Mutes voted at the 1878 World's Fair in Paris to accept Braille as the international writing system for the blind. The United States did not accept it until 1917.

In 1826, John Dix Fisher, a physician from Boston, Massachusetts, visited the National Institute for Blind Youth in Paris and was so impressed by what he saw there that he resolved to found a similar school in Boston. As a result of Fisher's efforts and the general mood of progressive humanitarian social reform that was sweeping New England at the time, the Massachusetts legislature voted in 1829 to establish the New England Asylum for the Blind—the first school for the blind in the United States. Fisher appointed Samuel Gridley Howe as its director.

In her history *The Imprisoned Guest: Samuel Howe and Laura Bridgman, the Original Deaf-Blind Girl,* Elisabeth Gitter gives an in-depth portrait of Howe, a man who was described by many as arrogant, vain, prideful, competitive, quick-tempered, defensive, overbearing, hungry for glory, a shrewd publicist and promoter, and generally unlikable. Howe's wife, the long-suffering Julia Ward Howe, stated that her husband was "incapable of enduring criticism or of profiting by it" and was also "much led by flattery." Charles Dickens called Howe a "cold-blooded fellow." Nevertheless, Howe was intelligent, determined, and had a genuine sense of empathy for the disadvantaged. In a letter to his friend Charles Sumner he wrote, "Every year I live brings closer to home the conviction that we must work for others & not for our own happiness." Howe's ambition for both himself and the Asylum for the Blind laid the foundation for what would become the world-famous Perkins Institution.

On a visit to the Paris institute, Samuel Howe was initially impressed with the school and pleased to see the blind students happily and diligently learning. However, after closer investigation, he found the school deeply disappointing. In an essay titled "Education of the Blind," published in the *North American Review* in 1833, Howe offered severe criticism of the Paris establishment in particular and of the other fledgling European institutes for the blind in general, stating that these European schools should be used only as cautionary examples; they represented everything that should be avoided in the founding of similar establishments in America. When Howe asked the authorities at the Paris institute how many of its graduates went on to support themselves with work, he was shocked at the response: "Not one in twenty." Incredulously, he remarked, "This is very like educating men for the almshouse," and he proceeded to condemn nearly every aspect of the school, from the impracticality of its teaching methods to its antiquated equipment to the amount of time wasted every day to its failure to address each individual student's particular talents to, finally, its self-satisfied atmosphere of showmanship, secrecy, and mystery.

> There pervades that establishment a spirit of illiberality, of mysticism, amounting almost to charlatanism... the process of education is not explained [to outside visitors], and the method of constructing some of the apparatus is absolutely kept a secret!... Those Institutions, endowed and supported by the governments, in general aim too much to show and parade; their object seems to be to teach the pupils to

perform such feats at the exhibition as will redound to the credit and glory of the government, rather than to their own good.

Howe's final slap for the European institutions for the blind was that the students were treated "too much as mere objects of pity; they are not taught to rely with confidence upon their own resources, to believe themselves possessed of the means of filling useful and active spheres in society." Howe's stated purpose in educating the blind was identical to Haüy's: to "enable them to pass their lives pleasantly and usefully in some constant occupation, which shall ensure to them a competent livelihood."

Gitter maintained that Howe's high ambition for his students was neither realistic nor practicable in the atmosphere of the era in which he was working. While Howe had none of the usual fear and revulsion at the sight of a blind person, many of his contemporaries—no matter how progressive or humanitarian they were—certainly did. Furthermore, Howe's goal for his blind students to be fully self-supporting once they left his school was unrealistic in an age of rapid industrialization.* More and more, the handicrafts—knitting, sewing, weaving— that the blind were taught were produced faster and with greater perfection by automated machines in the mills of Massachusetts.

By 1838 sixty students were enrolled at Howe's New England Asylum for the Blind. They learned to read raised letters, to write, to do arithmetic, geography, and most of the other subjects taught in regular schools for the sighted. Out of deference to the squeamishness of sighted visitors and school employees, students whose eyes were missing or disfigured wore wide green ribbons to hide the deformities. To raise financial support for the school, Howe staged public exhibitions

---

*In 2011, 63 percent of America's blind population of working age were unemployed. Thus, even now a "competent livelihood" is still a dream for the majority of the blind.

demonstrating the students' capabilities; the exhibitions were a great success, prompting many private citizens to donate funds and materials. The school rapidly became a celebrated cause in Boston society circles, and in 1839 it was renamed the Perkins Institution and Massachusetts Asylum for the Blind in honor of the shipping magnate Thomas H. Perkins, who donated a house for its use.

Howe's work brought him some renown in New England but nothing on the scale of the international fame that would visit him with the arrival of Laura Bridgman.

I am certain that I had never heard the name Laura Bridgman before I was forty-five years old. (I *had* heard the name Samuel Gridley Howe but could not attach it to anything in particular other than the readily recognizable name of his wife.) Very few people today seem to know who Laura Bridgman was. This is remarkable in light of the fact that, in her day, she was considered the most famous woman in the world other than Queen Victoria.

Bridgman was, as far as the records show, the first deaf-blind person to be successfully educated. Born in 1829 on a rural farm in Hanover, New Hampshire, she was, by her mother's account, a lively, intelligent, extremely curious child who had at eighteen months begun to "talk quite plain" and learn a few letters of the alphabet. But when she was two, she suffered a bout of scarlet fever that left her blind, deaf, and nearly devoid of the senses of taste and smell. Within a year, she had forgotten how to speak. (Her mother claimed that for a while after her illness, Laura repeated the words "Dark, dark" in puzzlement at her inability to see.) Laura was left with no form of communication other than crude gestures, and her early childhood resembled Helen Keller's in scope and emotion. Pressed from all sides by darkness and silence, she was often frustrated, unruly, and aggressive. Though her mother was loving, she was also busy with her other children and with the house and farm, and she must surely have been at a loss as to how to raise a child deprived of all but one of her five senses. Years later, Laura wrote lucidly of her life on the farm:

> I would cling to my mother so wildly and peevishly many times. I took hold of her legs or arms as she strode across the room. She acted so plain, as if it irritated her very much indeed. She scolded me sternly. I could not help feeling so cross and uneasy against her. I did not know any better. I never was taught to cultivate patience and mildness and placid[ity], until I came away from my blessed family at home.... My mother could not spell a single word to me with her fingers wishing me good night, nor good morning, [nor] Adieu, except that she gave me a most welcome kiss on my face. I did not know how to repay her for her welcome and cordiality.

As for communicating her desires:

> I offered my tiny hand to my mother, entreating her that she might know of my want for some thing to eat or drink. I stroked on my hand for some butter spread on a piece of bread. I could not assure her whatever I should like for a drink or nourishment, because I was incapable of making the deaf alphabet.... I used to make a sign for my dear mother that I wished to lie down on the bed. I nodded my head on my hand for that want of putting me immediately on the bed.

When Samuel Gridley Howe heard Laura's story, he saw in her an opportunity to experiment with the ongoing question of whether a blind-deaf child could be taught. Diderot had written about precisely this in his *Letter on the Blind.* "There is no communication between us and those born deaf, blind and mute. They grow, but they remain in a condition of mental imbecility. Perhaps they would have ideas, if we were to communicate with them in a definite and uniform manner from their infancy."* A child unexposed to sensory information, experiences, and ideas from the external world would provide Howe with an opportunity to study what in the human mind is innate and what is learned, the old Enlightenment question of the philosophy of the intellect, a question that still had not been answered entirely.

In 1837, when Laura was seven years old, Howe persuaded Bridgman's parents to let him take her to his asylum in Boston, and after working intensively with her for several months, he succeeded in making her understand the meaning and reason of language. In his *Ninth Annual Report of the Trustees of the Perkins Institution and Massachusetts Asylum for the Blind,* Howe described the epiphany:

> Hitherto, the process had been mechanical, and the success about as great as teaching a very knowing dog, a variety of tricks. The poor child had sat in mute amazement, and patiently imitated every thing her teacher did; but now the truth began to flash upon her—her intellect began to work—she perceived that here was a way by which she could herself make up a sign of any thing that was in her own mind, and show it to another mind, and at once her countenance lighted up with a human expression: it was no longer a dog, or parrot,—it was an immortal spirit, eagerly seizing upon a new link of union with other spirits!

Howe and the teachers he employed at Perkins taught Laura the manual alphabet of Charles de l'Épée. For a blind-deaf person such as Bridgman, the letters of the alphabet were formed with the fingers and pressed into the palm of the "listener's" hand.

---

*Most people deaf from a very young age are not, in fact, mute. They have functioning voices and can make sounds. They do not speak simply because they cannot hear and therefore cannot learn spoken language. Laura Bridgman could not speak but was not mute.

With Howe's writings about Laura and his frequent public exhibitions of her remarkable linguistic capabilities, the pair quickly captured the public imagination. In the 1840s, Howe's annual reports from the Perkins Institution—including private remarks that Laura made to her teachers as well as intimate details of her personal habits, her fastidiousness, her desire for affection and approbation—were in demand all over the United States and Europe. Newspapers and magazines began regularly printing sensational articles about the girl. A savvy publicist, Howe knew that the notoriety was good for the future of his school and used his storytelling ability to emphasize Bridgman's most admirable qualities—purity, sincerity, patience, determination—and thus appeal to the sentiments of his readers. In his *Eleventh Annual Report,* published in 1843, he wrote in his baroque style of Laura's transformed life at Perkins:

> She begins the day as merrily as the lark; she is laughing as she attires herself and braids her hair, and comes dancing out of her chamber as though every morn were that of a gala day; a smile and a sign of recognition greet everyone she meets; kisses and caresses are bestowed upon her friends and her teachers; she goes to her lesson, but knows not the word *task;* she gaily assists others in what they call housework, but which she deems play; she is delighted with society and clings to others as though she would grow to them, yet she is happy when sitting alone, and smiles and laughs as the varying current of pleasant thoughts passes through her mind; and when she walks out into the field, she greets her mother nature, whose smile she cannot see, whose music she cannot hear, with a joyful heart and a glad countenance; in a word, her whole life is like a hymn of gratitude and thanksgiving.

And, less cloyingly, in the *Ninth Report*:

The innate desire for knowledge, and the instinctive efforts which the Human faculties make to exercise their functions, are shown most remarkably in Laura. Her tiny fingers are to her as eyes, and ears, and nose, and most deftly and incessantly does she keep them in motion.... When she is walking with a person, she not only recognises [sic] everything she passes within touching distance, but by continually touching her companion's hands she ascertains what he is doing. A person walking across a room, while she had hold of his left arm, would find it hard to take a pencil out of his waistcoat pocket with his right hand, without her perceiving it.*

Finally, an excerpt from a letter that Howe wrote to the poet Mary Howitt†—and that she published in its entirety in her London magazine *Howitt's Journal of Literature and Popular Progress*—illustrates the spectacular mawkishness he was capable of in his portraits of Laura:

Is there not something very touching about it? A poor diseased child lived away up in the wild mountains of New Hampshire, her soul buried a thousand fathoms deep—so deep that no one could reach it or make a sign to it—under the burden of blindness, deafness, and mutism. But it was known that that soul was alive and struggling to get out into communion with other souls; and a hopeful man [himself] went to work to aid her, and toiled on for years, receiving at first a faint sign of recognition from below, and getting nearer and nearer, while people from all parts of the world looked eagerly on and uttered their words of encouragement; and when the child was raised by the hand and came out and walked with her fellows, all the people

---

*Laura's teachers claimed that she had an astonishing ability to judge people's moods and intentions; they believed she had a degree of extrasensory perception.

†Author of the poem "The Spider and the Fly."

raised a shout of joy, and poor little Laura Bridgman was raised into the human family with a heartier shout of welcome than a purple-born princess.

On his 1842 tour of America, Charles Dickens visited the Perkins Institution and was, not surprisingly, deeply moved by his meeting with Laura Bridgman. Hers was a case that would have fit ideally into one of his own novels. In his *American Notes for General Circulation*, Dickens quoted Howe's annual reports on Laura Bridgman at length, adding, "There are not many persons...who after reading these passages, can ever hear [Laura's] name with indifference." Of his own experience with Laura, he wrote:

> There she was before me; built up, as it were, in a marble cell, impervious to any ray of light, or particle of sound; with her poor white hand peeping through a chink in the wall, beckoning to some good man for help, that an Immortal soul might be awakened. Long before I looked upon her, the help had come. Her face was radiant with intelligence and pleasure. Her hair, braided by her own hands, was bound about a head, whose intellectual capacity and development were beautifully expressed in its graceful outline.... From the mournful ruin of such bereavement, there had slowly risen up this gentle, tender, guileless, grateful-hearted being.

Elisabeth Gitter suggested that for Dickens, as well as for the general public, "Laura mattered mostly as a metaphor...a kind of allegory...freed from her dark prison and summoned to life, she now had the power, through her example, to redeem the spiritually deaf and the morally blind." Upon publication of Dickens's *American Notes*, Laura Bridgman's fame exploded—hundreds of thousands of people on both sides of the Atlantic came to know and marvel at her story.

Now when Howe brought Laura on his traveling exhibitions, enormous crowds showed up for the spectacle. On the first Saturday of every month, the Perkins Institution was open to the public, and on those days the blind students demonstrated their various skills for visitors. As Laura's celebrity grew, the numbers of visitors to Perkins increased; on Saturday, July 6, 1844, eleven hundred people gathered to see Laura writing letters, reading books of raised type, threading fine needles with her tongue, and spelling sentences into her teacher's hand; they clamored for her autograph, pieces of her knitting and needlework, samples of her writing, and bits of her hair. All over America, little girls began poking their dolls' eyes out, tying green ribbons across them, and renaming them Laura.

Laura Bridgman became what the public wanted: an idealized, sentimentalized symbol of suffering tempered by goodness and hard work. She was an example of the power of the human spirit to overcome adversity. She was also a novelty in an age newly fascinated by celebrities and curiosities, a trend fostered and fueled by the advent of the high-speed printing press. Ernest Freeberg, in his history of Howe and Bridgman, *The Education of Laura Bridgman*, suggested that one explanation for Bridgman's fame was that she was a human aberration, "a freak of nature who captured the attention of a society that was hungry for spectacle," and that she happened to be living in a time when entrepreneurs like P. T. Barnum were turning human marvels into public entertainment. "The public's fascination with Laura Bridgman," he wrote, "might well be classified with their desire to see Barnum's exotic but 'scientific' curiosities, such as Tom Thumb and the Fiji Mermaid."*

---

*The Fiji Mermaid was billed as the mummified remains of a real-life mermaid—half human, half fish. It was, in fact, the head and torso of a baby monkey sewn to the rear half of a large fish and then covered so artfully with papier-mâché that it was entirely convincing. The Fiji Mermaid was destroyed in a fire just before the Wild Men of Borneo entered Barnum's fold.

Laura had no idea of the extent of the world's interest in her or of how much of her private daily life was exposed to the public, and she certainly had no control over it. Able to read only that which was available to her in raised type, she was not privy to most of the essays published about her. Her sense of self was strong enough, though, that she would probably have been annoyed and upset by the trespass on her privacy. Emotionally, Laura was extremely attached to and dependent on Howe, yet when Howe once opened a letter that was addressed to her, she was offended and firmly told him, "Doctor was wrong to open little girl's letters. Little girls open theirself."

The real Laura Bridgman was both more interesting and less angelic than Howe and Dickens led the public to believe. She was intelligent and had a very strong will, which at times she refused to curb to suit what Howe and the other teachers wanted of her. When she was instructed not to make loud and "disagreeable" noises with her unmodulated voice, she responded, "God gave me much voice!" Contrary to her public image, she was not always (in fact, not even often) a model, saintly child. Nor was she entirely "tender, gentle, and guileless." When a mouse got into her room, she managed to kill it by stomping on it. (Although this seems nearly impossible even for a person with the keenest eyesight, one of her teachers confirmed that the story was true.) She had fits of temper and more than once hit her adult teachers. She occasionally deceived them, several times stole food from other students, sometimes pushed, pinched, and bit people, and could be irritable, moody, and selfish. She was contemptuous of students who seemed to lack intelligence and she treated them imperiously. She was emotionally needy, had fits of nerves, and in her late teens became anorexic. She was, then, not unlike a lot of teenagers.

When Laura was eleven, Howe conceived of an experiment to isolate her from all religious ideas in an effort to determine whether notions of God came naturally to human beings or were instilled by others. He instructed her teachers to deflect any questions she had about God and religion. Inevitably exposed to religious notions through her contact with the other students, and having discovered the Bible in the Perkins Institution library, Laura was already inordinately curious about the subject.

Soon after Howe devised this scheme, he married Julia Ward, and they went abroad for eighteen months on their honeymoon. He was not present to oversee his own religious experiment with the girl, and he left her feeling utterly abandoned. Laura's mother—the only other person of extreme importance to her—was busy with five other children and the household demands of a farmer's wife and so had stopped responding to Laura's letters. At age fourteen, Laura was left to the care of a gifted but not exceptionally affectionate teacher, Mary Swift. The turmoil she was feeling, along with her confusion and bafflement at Swift's repeated deflections of her religious questions, began to manifest itself in unruly behavior and violent tantrums that Swift found increasingly difficult to subdue. In her teacher's journal, Swift gave an account of a battle of wills she and Laura had engaged in over a handkerchief. Swift always advised Laura to keep her handkerchief in her desk. On this particular day, Laura left it on top of her desk; Swift directed her to put it away, and Laura stubbornly put it in her lap instead. On Swift's insistence, Laura finally "lifted the lid very high, threw the handkerchief into the desk, and let it fall with such a noise as to startle all in the school-room. Her face was growing pale, and she was evidently getting into a passion." Swift directed her to take the handkerchief out of the desk and put it away properly. Laura "sat still awhile, and then uttered the most frightful yell that I ever heard. Her face was perfectly pale, and she trembled from head to foot."

As an evangelical Christian, Swift found it difficult to accept Howe's ban on religious instruction, particularly in the face of Laura's persistent question, "Why can I not know?" When a group of orthodox evangelical Christians came to the school, they ignored the request to refrain from religious discussion and gave Laura what amounted to a crash course in their beliefs. When Howe returned to Perkins and found Laura, who was no longer a child but a teenager, spouting evangelical dogma, he declared publicly that his project had been contaminated by "ignorant and selfish persons" and was therefore ruined. The blank slate that Laura had provided had been scrawled upon by interlopers; Howe was devastated by the failure.

With his project soured, disillusioned by both his own failure and Laura's glaring and seemingly sudden faults, he effectively turned against her. After years of pouring praise on her for the public's consumption, he now stated that his hopes for her had been disappointed "clearly because they were unreasonable" and because he had "overlooked" her "deranged constitution" and the "undue development" of her nervous system. In short, Howe maintained that Laura's flawed genetic inheritance and physical handicaps had warped her character and left her mentally and even intellectually defective.

Elisabeth Gitter argues, with much persuasive evidence, that Howe, who had a frequent habit of abandoning his own projects, had many complex personal reasons for feeling he couldn't continue his work with Laura Bridgman, including that he may have felt overshadowed and defined by Laura's fame and that "one way out was to claim that Laura was simply unfit for it." Which is, inarguably, the coward's way out. Gitter writes, "After 1844, he no longer thought her important." Realizing that the graduates of the Perkins Institution were in fact not able to support themselves with suitable work upon leaving the school, Howe seemed to turn against them too. (Although the public enjoyed seeing the Perkins students performing, the prejudice against them beyond its gates was still very strong. A local church that had hired the Perkins choir to sing regularly for its congregation soon told Howe that it had decided to "dispense with their services" because it didn't want to "subject any of the Society to unpleasant emotions," which tended to arise at the sight of the blind. Many of Howe's graduates wrote him letters requesting permission to return to the institution because they were failing to succeed in the outside world.)

Howe had stated firmly at the start of his career that the blind were no different from the sighted and that blindness was a superficial handicap, but after ten years of work at the Perkins Institution, he radically reversed his position. In his *Sixteenth Annual Report,* he claimed that his views had been modified by experience, and, in order to "unveil the shield of truth," he stated in emphatic uppercase letters: "THE BLIND, AS A CLASS, ARE INFERIOR TO OTHER PERSONS IN MENTAL POWER AND ABILITY." Contradicting in the extreme many of his earlier statements, Howe went on to insist that the senses, especially sight, are crucial to the development of the mind, and that people who were born blind or became blind due to illness were victims of poor heredity that left them inferior both mentally and physically. "Thus we see that the blind, as a class, do not labor under the disadvantage of want of sight alone, but that, as compared with others, they have less bodily health and vigor, and less mental power and energy." He described the blind boys who had recently entered Perkins as having "pale faces, stooping forms, puny limbs, feeble motions," and a "hesitating tread." Howe stated that his experiences with hundreds of blind people convinced him "that when children are born blind, or when they become blind early in life, in consequence of diseases which do not usually destroy the sight, the predisposing cause can be traced to the progenitors in almost all cases." Although Laura was rendered blind and deaf by scarlet fever, Howe suggested that her susceptibility to the disease and the resultant blindness derived from her slightly "scrofulous" and supposedly small-brained parents. (The parents naturally took umbrage.) And this was not simply a genetic failing he was positing; it was a moral one. "When men commit sin and violate the 'natural laws,' nature corrects them...she sends outward ailments as signs of inward infirmities." The moral transgressions—what Howe cryptically referred to as "sensual indulgences" and "hellish passions"—of the parents would be visited upon the children.

> The wit of man cannot devise a way of escape from the penalty of a violated law of nature; that not a single debauch, not a single excess, not a single abuse of any animal propensity, ever was or ever can be committed without more or less evil consequences; that sins of this kind are not and cannot be forgiven.... There will appear in the far-off and shadowy future the beseeching forms of little children,— some halt, or lame, or blind, or deformed, or decrepit,—crying, in speechless accents, "Forbear, for our sakes; for the arrows that turn aside from you are rankling in our flesh."

The report went on page after page in the same vein. There was a sense of personal injury in Howe's damning indictments of the blind. Despite all the progress that had been made over the past several thousand years, by 1850, the so-called father of the American blind had figuratively kicked them back to the Gospel according to Mark and its question "Master, who did sin, this man, or his parents, that he was born blind?"

It seems obvious to me that whatever Laura's emotional difficulties were, they had less to do with her physical disabilities than with the various traumas she had suffered in her young life. Consider the facts: As a very small child, she suddenly became unable to see, hear, or communicate and for five years afterward lived indeed like a household pet. At the age of seven, she was taken from the only place in the world that was familiar to her and delivered to an asylum a hundred and thirty miles away, where she found herself at the mercy of complete strangers for reasons utterly unknown to her; eighteen months passed before she met her mother again. She was used as a public socio-scientific experiment, constantly surveyed, corrected, manipulated, tested, and entreated to perform. She was more vulnerable than most children because of her sensory deprivations (she had a not unreasonable fear that she might fall off the edge of the floor, just as the earliest mariners feared they might sail off the edge of the flat earth), and the terror, confusion, and frustration that Laura Bridgman lived with must have been extremely difficult to cope with psychologically. One can only imagine the emotional riot that went on in her head. And the sole way for her to express her feelings civilly was to spell them out painstakingly with her fingers to those few people able to understand that language. (Laura's own parents never properly learned the manual alphabet.) Her emotional difficulties were surely not caused by her blindness but by the upheaval she had endured.

Toward the end of her life, Annie Sullivan stated that she had "always believed Laura Bridgman to be intellectually superior to Helen Keller." Keller herself said that if Bridgman had had Sullivan as a teacher, "she would have outshone me." Yet despite her remarkable intellect, following her brief period of celebrity, Laura Bridgman lived out the rest of her years in obscurity, abandoned by her teacher and by society, a lifelong resident of the Perkins Institution, monotonously doing needlework and reading embossed books, a shut-in no less than she had been as a child on the farm in rural New Hampshire.

## The Blind

*Consider them, my soul; they are truly horrific!*
*Similar to mannequins; vaguely ridiculous;*
*Terrible, strange as sleepwalkers*
*Darting, one knows not where, their shadowy globes.*

*Their eyes, from which the divine spark is gone,*
*How they gaze afar, raised up*
*To the sky; never do they gaze at the pavement beneath them,*
*Dreamily bending their heavy heads.*

*They pass this way through endless night,*
*That brother of eternal silence. Oh, city!*
*While around us you sing, laugh and bellow,*

*Taking pleasure in the atrocity,*
*Look! I drag myself too! but more stupefied than they,*
*I say: What are they seeking in the sky, all these blind people?*

—Charles Baudelaire; translated by Ellen Mahoney Sawyer with
Frances Papazafiropoulos

# Navigation

The International Institute for Social Entrepreneurs,[*] the newest offshoot of Braille Without Borders, is located in southern India, in the state of Kerala, some eleven or so miles outside the city of Trivandrum in the little village of Nemom Po. The village is a scattering of brick houses and shacks built along a network of one-lane roads that wind through a vast, dense jungle of coconut, mango, and banana trees. The small campus of the institute lies at the edge of a freshwater lake called Vellayani.

One evening during my first week at the institute, in January of 2009, I stepped out of the office building and found Sabriye Tenberken standing on a footpath in the dark with Basant, a blind Indian computer expert. The only light on the path came from a tepid bulb above the door of the dining room, just beyond where they stood. That the light was feeble made no difference to them. They didn't need it. But I did. Without it I would not have known that there were three or four fruit bats appearing and swiftly disappearing just inches above their heads, swerving and fluttering and repulsively large. The bats had heads the size of a Chihuahua's and their wingspans were half as wide

---

[*]In 2012 the name of the institute was changed to kanthari.

as an open golf umbrella. They were so big they did not dart or flit as normal bats do; instead, they lurched. It was their blindness that led them to fly so close to an object, and their sharp hearing that steered them away again.

Sabriye, wearing a yellow baseball cap and her ever-present portable Braille computer on a strap across her chest, was holding Basant's wrist and drawing on his palm with her fingertip. She was teaching him the layout of the IISE campus, the shape of the dorms; she was even detailing a few small outbuildings that had yet to be built. "And here is the jetty," she said, "and here the dock at the lake's edge, and here the swimming pool, although none of that is there yet." She was teaching a blind man the shape of things that didn't exist, which is not fundamentally different from teaching a blind man the shape of things that *do* exist. Whether the objects were there or not, Basant would henceforth retain their precise configuration and location in his mind, just as Sabriye had done.

"The shape of the dining room and auditorium building is that of a whale, and the shape of the amphitheater is like the number nine," Sabriye said. "Do you know what a nine looks like?"

Blind from birth, Basant did not know what a nine looked like. Sensing my presence beside her—and I mean by this that she sensed in her eerie way *my* particular presence and not just the presence of some anonymous human being—Sabriye turned toward me and asked me how one could best describe the shape of a 9. I thought about it. "How about a snake that has turned the front part of its body backward to examine its own midsection?"

Basant didn't know exactly what a snake looked like. This surprised me, for he was a local man, and the area around Lake Vellayani is, like the entire state of Kerala, not just full of large fruit bats but full of many very large snakes as well. I drew a 9 on Basant's palm. He couldn't make sense of it. I asked permission to draw the number on his forehead, which seemed to me an excellently flat, smooth, sensitive slate through which he could surely feel and thereby perceive the shape of a small figure. He gave me permission, and as I drew the 9, he giggled uproariously.

Basant is a large, polite, extremely intelligent man with a head of thick black hair. He has long hair growing out of his ears. Like many Indians, he eschews a knife and fork and eats with his hands. Giggling is one of his salient characteristics. His giggling is high-pitched and triggered by anything remotely risqué or unexpected, and when he giggles, he raises his right shoulder, places his chin firmly upon it with his mouth pinched shut and twisted off to the left, and lifts one hand to hide his face. It is the giggle of a nervous, delighted, slightly scandalized ten-year-old girl. He speaks English with a plummy upper-class British-Indian accent and the interjectory ejaculations of Henry Higgins. To wit: "Indeed, Rose, indeed," and "Oh, quite!," and "Too true!"

Basant, who happens to be a chess prodigy, began his working life as an operator in a public telephone kiosk. Such kiosks, approximately twice the size of the conventional enclosed public phone booth, are found all over India. "I was sitting in that little booth all day, like in a prison," he told me. "I was just doing nothing but reading books six hours a day and dialing phone calls. I felt I was wasting my time. And the people I met just humored me. They didn't take me seriously."

When I asked him what sort of books he read, he said quickly, "*Robinson Crusoe*. I liked that tremendously."

It made sense that a story about a castaway on the Island of Despair would appeal to a blind man trapped in a phone booth with no apparent exit.

Basant met some customers who were well versed in computer technology, and they informed him about various computer programs, including programs that could help sharpen one's chess skills. He purchased one of these programs, rapidly improved his game, and began winning chess titles. (Chess pieces for the blind have pegs at their bottoms, rather like cribbage pegs; each peg fits into a small hole drilled into the center of each square, and this holds them steady at the touch of blindly searching fingers.) At the time of our meeting, Basant was the chess champion of the state of Kerala. His experience with the chess programs inspired his interest in other software, especially software geared toward the blind. He was now expert with JAWS and Orca, the speech-synthesizer programs that read aloud to the listener whatever text appears on the computer screen, thus enabling blind users to operate conventional computers.

Eager to see how a blind man played chess, I had challenged Basant to a game earlier that day. I marveled at the delicacy with which his large fingers identified the various pieces, at the skill and precision with which he moved each to its next destination and nimbly inserted it into its hole, and at how, after each move I made, he felt what I had done with his right hand, touched the few pieces around it, and kept the layout of the board in his mind. And then, almost before it had begun, the game was abruptly over, and I was left sitting with my mouth agape at how quickly he had beaten me. Seven moves apiece was the extent of the match.

"Tell me, Basant," I said now, "how bad was my game?"

"Not at all bad, Rose. Not bad," he said in his transparently well-mannered way.

"Come now, Basant, you can tell me. How bad am I at chess?"

"No, not too bad at all."

"Basant?"

He ducked his head. "Yes?"

"Don't bullshit me. How bad was my chess game?"

All that was visible of Basant's eyes was a thin sliver of white between his permanently half-closed lids. He lifted his shoulder, placed his chin upon it, and giggled out of the corner of his mouth with his left hand screening his face like a geisha's paper fan. Eventually he sobered up and mustered the courage to tell me: "Well, I must say you fall far short, Rose. *Far* short."

Several months later, when I reminded Basant of our chess game and asked him if he remembered it, he recalled in exact sequence all fourteen moves and began to repeat them back to me. I said, "Thank God I am not a blind genius burdened by the sequence of moves of every chess game I have ever played."

This triggered an unusually prolonged fit of giggling.

Memory is a crucial skill for the blind. Without vision to assist it, the memory works overtime, situating and defining many pieces of information that cannot easily be checked twice. After Sabriye typed up the schedule of classes and staff meetings for an entire week, she automatically retained the schedule in her memory, recalling with ease the time and location of every event that would take place over the next seven days. She had the same skill with her physical surroundings. Her knowledge and memory of the location of every tree, pothole, door, and light switch in her environs was truly astonishing. One day two years before, while I was sitting with Sabriye in her office at the Braille Without Borders farm in Tibet, a strong wind came up, and an attic door above us began to bang. Sabriye jumped up from her desk, hurried out into the hallway without her white cane, clambered up a nearly vertical ladder, pulled the door shut, and hopped back down, all in less time than it would have taken a sighted person.

After saying good-bye to Basant that evening, Sabriye invited me to see where she and Paul lived. Their house was a four-minute walk from the campus. The institute was separated from the local population by a surrounding wall and a large iron gate manned at all times by an Indian guard. When we went out through the school's front gate, the guard in his uniform stood up so nervously and abruptly that I half expected him to give us a military salute. We turned right and set off down a narrow road that led through a coconut grove. As we moved away from the lights of the school, the road quickly became dark—so dark I could make nothing out, could not see my own hand when I held it before my face. I told Sabriye that I could see nothing and therefore would be of no assistance getting her to her house, and as soon as I said it, I realized what a foolish statement it was. She hooked her arm through mine and said with mild irony, "I know how to get there."

Though I knew how well Sabriye navigated and knew how many times she had been on this road, I was a little nervous. The road narrowed quickly, and eventually the surface changed from pavement to dirt. It was riddled with potholes and many small stones. I had walked here once already and knew that a family of mean turkeys lived not far up the road, turkeys who had a propensity to chase human beings and even try to bite them. And there were dogs here, mangy, starved-looking wild dogs with staring black eyes and sharp teeth. And I was certain we had a flock of those creepy bats following us—I could fairly feel them stirring the air above my head. "I really can't see a thing," I said.

"Don't worry. I know every inch of this road." Sabriye explained that she couldn't really get turned around here because of the breeze that generally blew in off the lake. If she could feel the breeze on her cheek, she knew where the lake was, and if she knew where the lake was, she knew in which direction she was headed. The same was true of the sun: If she knew what time it was and felt the sun shining at a certain angle on her face, she knew what direction she was facing.

I asked Sabriye what prevented her from walking into the barbed-wire fences and coconut trees that lined the road.

"I can sense them. It's a kind of echo that they make. I know when an object is in front of me."

"How could a barbed-wire fence make an echo?" I said.

She assured me that it somehow did, that she could not just hear but feel its presence like a vibration, and that she had been on this road so many times that she knew where every object and pitfall was. I could hear the tip of her white cane occasionally tapping the earth. Three years before, when I visited her in Tibet, Sabriye had explained to me that the white cane was useful not simply because it came in contact with obstacles before its user did but also because the sound the cane made from one situation to the next revealed a great deal of information. The sort of echo the tapping cane made would tell the user what kind of space she was in. She could determine from the quality of the echo not just that a street was lined with houses but whether the houses were made of stone or of wood, could tell whether a street was bordered by trees or shrubbery, degrees of subtlety that could come only with long hours of practice. Some blind people don't like to use the white cane, feeling that it too loudly brands them as blind and helpless. Sabriye, though, was the cane's strongest advocate. She carried her cane wherever she went. Sighted people unfamiliar with the purpose of the white cane sometimes asked her in her travels if she was a shepherd, or if the stick was a piece of skiing equipment or perhaps a device for detecting land mines.

We walked silently for a bit, listening to the sound of our own footsteps on sandy gravel, the rustling of creatures in the underbrush at the side of the road, the occasional hoot or wail of a bird. Kerala's darkness of night—the deepest darkness I've ever experienced anywhere—could not completely still the impulses of its remarkably robust wildlife, a wildlife I had begun to familiarize myself with with some alarm. Before coming here I had done a little research about the area and was not heartened to read this:

> All the major venomous species of snakes found in India are also found in Kerala. Kerala is recognized as having a major problem

with snakebite. The five common poisonous snakes found in Kerala are Indian Cobra, King Cobra, Russel's Viper, Saw-scaled Viper and Krait. Out of these, Indian Cobra, Russel's Viper, Saw-scaled Viper and Krait are the most dangerous, since King Cobra usually habits in dense forests and hence rarely comes in contact with humans.

I understood this to mean that in Kerala, there was no question but that I would come in contact with four out of these five species of venomous snake, to say nothing of Kerala's many species of nonvenomous snake, which I was no more eager to meet.

Trailing slightly behind Sabriye, lightly tugged along by the crook of her elbow, I said a bit breathlessly, "We won't meet any snakes, will we?"

Sabriye did not exactly assure me that we wouldn't meet a snake but said that if we did, it would probably be a rat snake, and that would be all right because rat snakes were not poisonous and therefore not dangerous. "But rat snakes are big," she added. "And if they bite you, you bleed a lot."

"I *do?*"

"Yes, but usually you don't die."

I remained silent after that. I didn't want to hear any more. I was by now familiar with Sabriye's nonchalance, her directness, her sense of humor, and her habit of extreme understatement, all of which I generally appreciated. But that night I struggled to contain my feelings of reluctance as she dragged me stumbling up the road.

We arrived at the house, and Sabriye led me inside and set about making me a cup of tea. The house was typical of many in the area, a surprisingly modern construction probably not more than ten years old, two stories high, with a well-appointed kitchen, a dining room/living room, two bedrooms, two bathrooms, a driveway, and a carport—a brightly painted, suburban sort of house in the middle of a coconut jungle.

We sat at a table drinking our tea, talking about her and Paul's plan for the school year ahead. I noticed that Sabriye's bare ankles were flecked with mosquito bites. The yellow baseball cap on her head sat slightly askew and her long blond hair was a bit jumbled beneath it. As attractive as Sabriye is, her appearance is probably the last thing on her mind. Most days she dresses casually in jeans and a T-shirt. When she dresses up for an occasion, the transformation is stunning. Tonight she looked tired but happy.

Sabriye and Paul Kronenberg had been working nonstop for several years to make the IISE in Kerala a reality. The first students had already arrived, and the rest would be arriving within a few days. I could feel Sabriye's satisfaction and excited anticipation. Even at her most relaxed, she has an intense way of speaking—the words spill out of her with an urgency and a clarity of enunciation that grabs the listener by the earlobes. This, combined with the musical strength of her voice, makes it nearly impossible not to pay attention to what she's saying.

That night she spoke of their goals here, their desire to help other blind and socially motivated people realize their dreams of improving the lives of others, of making a contribution to society. She told me that her parents were artistic and that when she was growing up they always had a lot of artistic people in the house, which made for a rather chaotic atmosphere. "There were a lot of big talkers around us. They didn't do much, but they talked a lot. My parents started a school for creative arts in Germany. They opened their house to the public, and that opened my mind to another way of looking at things. When I went blind, I went from being popular to being an outcast. Nobody wanted to sit next to me in school. I became very angry. There is a word in German: *wut*. It expresses an anger like outrage. It's a productive kind of anger."

Sabriye referred—as she often does—to the high school for the blind that she attended in Marburg, Germany, to the impact it had on her, and to the confidence she learned there. "The special thing about that school," she said, "was that the teachers didn't overprotect the students. They said, 'You may be blind but you still have a talent and a brain, and you have dignity.' The important thing was confidence, and how to deal with your own blindness in a humorous way."

Beyond the walls of that school, Sabriye faced discrimination. Even her friends told her she couldn't accomplish much because of her blindness. In Germany, the legally blind are entitled to a government stipend of five hundred dollars a month. Sabriye felt that the blind didn't need subsidies, that all they really needed was equal rights. "Blind German people study at university," she said. "They have degrees in everything. But seventy percent of them are unemployed because of prejudice. People don't like change. The status quo is comfortable. German people are very conservative, and the German blind are still suffering from the attitudes of the Third Reich. We are still seen as worthless, as a burden to society. It's all still there. Younger Germans are interested in these issues but the older ones are happy to just sit and drink their beer."

On the advice of one of her teachers, when Sabriye finished university, she decided to go into development work. She wanted to travel and be useful to others, to use her talents and get her hands dirty. She approached the Red Cross and Caritas to see if they would employ her; their response was *Don't do this to us. We don't have insurance to cover you.* "Sighted people tell the blind, 'You cannot do it,' but they only say this because *they* cannot do it. My feeling was, if they won't send me into the field, I'll start my own organization and send myself. So I'm blind. So *what?*"

Once Paul and Sabriye had gotten the Braille Without Borders school in Tibet on its feet, they wanted to start a center for people who had what Sabriye called "big dreams," a center for the blind where no one would say no to their ambitions of social entrepreneurship.

They chose India because it is geographically central to the world's developing countries, from which the student body would be drawn, and because the Indian health care system is good, and because India's population is relatively well educated. The participants in the program would spend a year learning the skills necessary to found and run a not-for-profit organization: management, leadership, communication, budgeting, fund-raising, bookkeeping, public speaking, writing, advertising, marketing, hiring, and computer proficiency. They wanted not just to teach these skills but to create a think-tank where the exchange of ideas among the participants would be the guiding force. They would accept sighted people as well as blind, as long as the applicants had conviction and strong intellectual social vision. They had hired some twelve or thirteen people to help them run the program, including housekeepers and a kitchen staff. The student body for the coming year would number twenty-four in all. They would live together in the dormitory, two to a room—women on the second floor, men on the first. This was a very different arrangement from the school Paul and Sabriye were running in Tibet and would be a new challenge for them. Tibetan children required one kind of attention and one set of guidelines; blind and visually impaired adults from thirteen different countries required something entirely different. The IISE was a bigger property, and the cost of transporting, feeding, housing, and educating the participants would be roughly 6,500 euros per student; the total cost of running the institute would be 170,000 euros that year.

Eventually Paul joined us at the kitchen table. He is a tall, slender, blond-haired, blue-eyed Dutchman with a film star's evenly sculpted features. See him from the corner of your eye and for a moment you might think he's Ralph Fiennes. An extremely hardworking, passionate, and dedicated man, Paul has a zeal for their projects that is palpable. He is a storyteller who feels things deeply, shows his emotions freely, and can be moved to cry by a particularly poignant story—his own or someone else's. Paul confessed that night that he'd been working so hard and sleeping so little he had lost weight. I saw that; I saw that his clothes hung more loosely on his frame than they had in Tibet, and that his eyes were reddish from lack of sleep.

Paul's ambitions and talents are varied, but he is particularly knowledgeable and passionate about architectural design and its relationship to the natural environment. It was he who designed most of the buildings on the Braille Without Borders farm in Shigatse, Tibet, and with results that are extremely pleasing to the eye. Having raised enough money through grants and donations to buy the land here at the edge of the lake and fund the construction of the institute, Sabriye and Paul felt strongly that their first task was to design a campus that was as environmentally friendly, cost-effective, and energy efficient as possible. They were as concerned and idealistic about the future of the earth's ecology as they were about the future of humanity—concerns and ideals that obviously go hand in hand. Paul said, "We feel that when we try to change things for blind people worldwide, we should also work on changing something about the environmental approach. If you set up a project like this, you also have to build it in an environmentally friendly way."

Paul and Sabriye were inspired in part by the British architect Laurie Baker, who went to northern India in 1945 to build practical, low-cost hospitals for lepers. Baker believed that poor people didn't have to live in poor conditions, and he demonstrated that it didn't take a lot of money to build a pleasant house. He became acquainted with Mohandas Gandhi, who embraced Baker's approach, and when most foreigners were asked to leave India after independence, Gandhi invited Baker to stay and continue his work. In the span of sixty years, Baker designed and built many houses and public buildings around the city of Trivandrum—practical, low-cost, and aesthetically pleasing structures. Rather than impose modern, foreign architectural methods on his constructions, Baker embraced the indigenous traditional practices and simply modified them.

"Baker's first concern was low cost," Paul said. "But the style he chose was also good for the environment. We followed that style because we want to show people that it's possible to live in harmony with the environment."

The first rule of this sort of construction was that the building materials should come from within a fifteen-mile radius, which decreased not only transportation costs but also energy consumption and the resultant pollutants. The four main campus buildings at the IISE were made of recycled materials and locally manufactured brick and tile. Paul and Sabriye deliberately installed air-conditioning only in the computer lab, where it was necessary to keep the equipment from overheating. Otherwise, all the buildings were cooled in a natural process: Portions of the walls of the campus buildings were constructed in the *jali* design, in which the bricks were arranged to make a pattern of gaps in the wall, allowing air to enter at the lower parts of the building, rise naturally, and then exit through similar gaps at the top of the building, causing a cooling circulation and giving the buildings a pretty, whimsical aspect that no other buildings in the area possessed. In addition, all the campus buildings were graced with balconies and large windows.

Paul began to speak about toilets and waste management. "In the West, we use water toilets," he said. "It's not a very environmentally friendly method. Ecosan is a movement aimed at getting rid of our waste in a more efficient and less harmful way. If you mix urine with feces you get a worse smell than if the two are kept separate. The ecosan toilet separates them."

The toilet in my dorm room, like all the toilets at the institute, was an ecosan toilet. I had seen for myself how the separation worked. The toilet bowl was, in a sense, two bowls—smaller at the front, larger at the rear. If you sat on the toilet seat, a lever was pressed that opened a drain at the bottom of the front bowl of the toilet where the urine was collected. The urine, without added water, would drain to a tank outside the dorm building. When you stood up, that pipe would close so that when you flushed the toilet, the water was prevented from escaping through it and would carry only the feces out the back side of the toilet to a separate bio-gas tank, where it would be transformed into fuel.

"Urine added with a little bit of water can be used to water trees and plants, and it acts as a fertilizer," Paul said. "And the feces is working to create a source of energy. So, every time you go to the toilet you feel good because you're adding benefit."

Sabriye snickered at the idea.

"We hope that we can find manufacturers within India who'll start to make these toilets."

They were hoping to purchase two windmills for the campus in order to generate their own electricity and were also planning to harness solar energy. "We want a solar-powered boat for our participants to use on the lake. One drop of gasoline pollutes billions of liters of water, and a gas engine is noisy. A solar boat is quiet, doesn't pollute, and runs on the energy of the sun."

Whenever he makes a statement like this, Paul presents his hands palms upward to show the sense and simplicity of it all and then he looks you in the eye and smiles like a man who has just won the lottery. "Our solar boat will be the first ever in Kerala."

"So you're not just educating blind people," I said. "Your entire way of life is a kind of example of how we can save the environment and ensure a sustainable future."

Perhaps anticipating skepticism, Sabriye said, "People scoff at us all the time. They tell us we're too idealistic, that our dreams are beyond our reach, that one person can't change the world. One person *can't* change the world, of course, but many people working together can. If one person shows another what can be done and that one shows another and each one takes a responsibility for his own way of life and does his part, the world *does* change."

"We built a concrete housing system for the storage of rainwater," Paul said. "We didn't really need it, because we have the lake water, but we did it to show people that you can collect rainwater in dry places and store it underground for later use. It's an example."

Sabriye laughed. "The local people saw the storage tanks and were convinced we were going to use them to store alcohol."

"Alcohol is taboo here," Paul said and went on to explain that the local people living near the school kept a curious and sometimes suspicious eye on their progress as the institute was being built. Not sure what to make of this foreign presence and its unprecedented construction in their dozy little community, the locals seemed to feel envy, fear, and excitement. When the peripheral wall of the campus was constructed for privacy, some neighbors tried to break it down, protesting that part of the land it was enclosing belonged to them. Paul had had to do a great deal of explaining and appeasing to keep the peace. "I tried to get them to see that we can all work together and that everyone could benefit from our presence. I told them, 'The fact that we're here could be good for you. For example, we can buy the vegetables you grow in your gardens for our kitchen,' but they were wary."

The area was ruled by labor unions with an extremely territorial grasp. By law, any goods delivered to the institute had to be unloaded by union workers only. "You can't even unload deliveries on your own private property," Paul said with exasperation. "You have to let the union men in and pay them to do it." Whenever the union men saw a truck heading down the road toward the institute, they ran after it to ensure that the job of unloading it was theirs. If private individuals tried to unload the goods themselves, the union men could become aggressive, even violent. "We've had plenty of difficulties, but we're so lucky to be here," Paul said.

In the subsequent months, I would lose count of the number of times Paul Kronenberg cited his good fortune in life, and every time he did, it struck me anew. I had never met a person who felt so lucky with his lot and expressed that feeling so often, and I'd certainly never met anyone who felt lucky to be spending his life in the constant service of others.

"One thing we're very concerned with is the development of affordable technology for the blind," Sabriye said. "Most good technology is really expensive or not even available for people in poor countries. Who in the developing world can afford a Perkins Brailler? Who can afford a Marburg Brailler? Nobody! They cost two hundred and fifty dollars apiece! The less expensive ones are no good. We use a machine in Tibet that's a shitty version of the Marburg machine. It falls apart if you press on it too hard. It's not a pleasure to write with that machine. Paul is a mechanical engineer. He's designing a Braille machine that's light and small enough to fit in your pocket. We want to get input from our participants here to create new technology for the blind that's high-quality and low-cost."

"There's a lot you want to do," I said.

"Yes," Sabriye said, turning her blue eyes to me and shrugging her shoulders, "and why not?"

As I got up to leave that night, Sabriye gave me a flashlight to use on the walk home. I said good night, went out to the road, and set off at a brisk jog to get the return trip over with as quickly as I could. Similar to the way Sabriye wagged the tip of her white cane before her, I shone the beam of light from side to side as I ran, looking for any threat. The sides of the road were littered with palm fronds and bits of coconut shells. I hoped that the sound of my heavy footsteps would scare off the snakes and turkeys, and I thought that if some snake was chasing me, he wouldn't be able to catch me if I was running. (When I finally saw my first rat snake, I realized that even if I sprinted, I could not outrun it. I had been walking on the main road near Vellayani Temple amid scores of people heading home on foot after work when I turned my head and saw an enormous, sinister mustard-green snake the thickness of an engorged fire hose wriggling vigorously toward me across an empty lot. The snake, nine or ten feet long, was moving at what I can describe only as an urgent pace, as if being chased. It slowed suddenly when it reached the hot pavement and then glided its way idly across the crowded road amid the feet of the pedestrians. Appalled, not quite believing my eyes, I stopped in my tracks. But when I saw that the snake evoked no reaction whatever from the Indian crowd— the people stepped blithely, some of them shoeless, over or around this slithering, glistening mass of muscle—I began walking again toward the snake with my heart in my throat. I continued walking because I suffer the sin of pride; I am loath to reveal that I am afraid of a physical threat. I simply refused to be the only person in the crowd with her palms to her cheeks screaming, *Mother of God, don't you people see that the biggest, grossest snake in the world is about to wrap itself around your ankles?* So, I carried on, doing what the Indians did. I made sure to show no emotion whatever, although every inch of my being was recoiling in primal disgust and fear. The snake disappeared into the long grass on the other side of the road but stayed horribly in my mind for days afterward.)

The state of Kerala suffers much the same poverty, overpopulation, pollution, disorder, and general social mayhem that the rest of India suffers, but Kerala has the added hardships of a rampant wildlife and an overbearing climate. To my mind, Kerala is *extremely* India. When people asked me where I was going to be in India and I responded,

"Kerala," they inevitably said, "Oh, Kerala is beautiful!" Kerala may be beautiful, but I am unable to see the beauty. I have never been in an environment so antithetical to my idea of pleasing, so far from my concept of hospitable, so far from my notion of beautiful. Much of my discomfort arose from the heat and humidity. On most days in Trivandrum, the temperature was about 92 degrees, with a humidity of 88 percent. This is nothing like the heat of Egypt or Greece or even Death Valley or the Dead Sea. In those hot places the heat is sharp and clean, like an elegant knife blade that cuts you in a mercifully swift and tidy fashion so that by nightfall you forget you've been wounded. Here, the heat is not just constant but incontinent. It is pervasive and sloppy, suffocating as a pillow placed in boiling palm oil and then pressed firmly over the face. It seeps into every crevice and corner and adheres to whatever it touches. It creeps into the mind. It fouls the atmosphere. In Trivandrum, after one's clothes have been hanging in the closet for a few days, they begin to smell powerfully musty. There were days at the IISE when the afternoon heat and humidity were so great that I felt I could not breathe in my room, and at those times, I headed out to the balcony in a pathetic, reflexive way, telling myself, *Go outside, it will be better there.* But unlike the thin air of Tibet, which was always the same, outside or in, the air in Trivandrum was always worse outside. Outside, there seemed to be less air, and the air on my balcony usually smelled like broiled urine because the outhouse of the family of five who lived just over the school's boundary wall was situated extremely close to my bedroom. And the air was often dosed with smoke from the coconut shells and palm fronds and assorted domestic waste the local village families were in the habit of burning outside their huts.

In Trivandrum, the sky always had a yellowish tint, even on the clearest, sunniest day, and a great weariness seemed to hang over everything. The buildings along the main road going into the city looked senile and decrepit. And everywhere I looked in Trivandrum, I was, strangely, reminded of death. Nothing looked fresh. On an overcast day, even the clouds looked sad and exhausted and seemed to droop onto the tops of the buildings. The tropical birds didn't sing a pretty melody in the way of birds that I was familiar with. Instead, they shrieked and howled like women being stabbed with a carving knife. They wailed and whooped as though irate and besieged. Even the local chipmunks had a savage streak. When angered, they raised their tails at you in a threatening way and barked maniacally, and you knew for certain that if one of those creatures managed to get within an inch of your face, it would surely claw your eyes out. In the morning, carrion crows by the score made sharp, extremely loud retching sounds. Sometimes they were so loud I had to close the windows in order to hear myself think above the racket.

People always said that Lake Vellayani, which abutted the school, was beautiful. To my eyes, the only thing about it that was beautiful was that it was a wide-open space, a merciful break in the claustrophobia of coconut, banana, and mango trees. Also, it did allow a breeze to sweep through the west side of the campus. When I first looked at the lake, I thought, *Is it* really *a lake? Or is it just a swamp?* The lake water was an opaque mud-brown. There were snakes in it and water rats and leeches, so I heard, and frogs that were frighteningly large. And where the lake was not covered with lily pads the size of manhole covers, it was blanketed with water bugs pullulating on the surface. And although I don't think I ever saw one, I was told there were mongooses there. I knew that the mongoose is a red-eyed, foxlike thing with a thousand carpet tacks for teeth. When someone informed me that the mongoose is our friend because he eats cobras, all I could think was that if a mongoose is bold enough and clever enough to eat a cobra, he's clever enough to eat me. One day I saw at the edge of the lake an enormous brown ratlike thing with a wrinkled, smashed-in sort of face, like a Chinese shar-pei. I had never seen such a creature before and never did determine what it was. At certain times of the day dragonflies by the dozen hazed the surface of the lake. The dragonfly is a beautiful insect, but in numbers like this, they concerned me. I would see these flickering, flashing droves and think, *You could be overpowered by them and get your nose chewed off.*

I sound like a fearful person. I am not, truly, but I am a firm believer in one novel thing at a time and everything in its place. Kerala's wildlife was ever present, seemed to come at me all at once, even into my bedroom, multiplying before my eyes. It was attention grabbing and *distracting.* In her poem "This Is Disgraceful and Abominable," the poet Stevie Smith barked at her readers, "Animals are animals and have their nature / And that's enough, it is enough, leave it alone." Gladly I would leave it alone, if only it would leave me alone.

I ran all the way back to the gate of the school, deposited Sabriye's flashlight in her office, and returned to my room at the end of the dormitory. The dormitory rooms were connected by an outside walkway that was covered with a kind of porch roof, rather like the design of a motel. My bedroom was a pleasant, comfortable, square space with yellow walls and red terra-cotta tiles on the floor. It was appointed with a small armoire, a desk, two chairs, and a bunk bed set against one wall. There was a large electric fan affixed to the ceiling and two smaller fans that had been mounted on the walls, one just above the top bunk, where I slept. The bathroom was utilitarian but clean and bright. A screen door opened onto a small balcony that looked out over the rear of the building to the plot of coconut and mango trees just beyond the school's wall, and a large window on the opposite wall opened over the outdoor staircase that led down to the ground floor. There were screens on the windows. I had everything I needed.

I put on the light and the ceiling fan and sat at my desk, preparing to make some notes before going to bed. As I was reaching for my notebook, all the lights on the campus went out. I had been informed that scheduled half-hour power cuts would occur every evening in this part of Trivandrum, a blunt energy-saving measure geared to ensure there was enough electricity to go around. Though the area looked like a wild jungle to me, there were thousands upon thousands of people living around the lake, and the supply of electricity was obviously not meeting the demand. When the lights go out at night in Vellayani, whatever room you happen to be in goes not just dark but completely black. It is like having a canvas sack pulled over your head.

I patted my hands around my desk, searching for my cell phone, thinking to use its illuminated screen as a way to find my own flashlight, which was still at the bottom of my suitcase. In my clumsy search, I smashed a water glass, dumping water over the pages of my open notebook. I cut the heel of my palm on a shard of the broken glass and failed to find the cell phone, although I knew it was within arm's reach. I could feel the sticky wetness of blood running down my fingers. I stood up and went across the floor in the direction of the bathroom with my hands held out in front of me to protect myself from what I couldn't see. I had occupied this room for only three days and was still not entirely familiar with its contours. My hands met the wall. As I slid my bare feet across the floor in the direction of the bathroom, I smashed my big toe badly on the foot of the armoire. Limping now, I felt my way along the wall, entered the bathroom, moved to where I knew the sink was, and in groping for the faucets, I knocked my toothbrush and comb into the open toilet beside the sink. I knew they had fallen into the toilet by the taunting little tinkling sound they made against the porcelain. Eager to wash my bloody hand, I turned the faucets on. No water. (I wasn't yet aware that on this campus, no electricity meant no water pump and often no water.) In taking my hand away from the faucet I knocked something else onto the floor but wasn't sure what it was. I crouched down, patted the floor, couldn't find anything, and as I moved to get up again I banged my head on the sink. I turned from the sink, shuffled to the wall beside the toilet, ran my fingers down it until I found the toilet-paper dispenser, and wrapped my hand with paper. With timid, mincing little steps and my hands held up before my face (which, I realized after a while, was tensed into a grimace of self-defense; not only that, but I was walking with my head bowed so fearfully deeply that my chin was literally pressed against my chest), I caromed back to the desk chair and sat there in the mounting heat. (No electricity, no ceiling fan. And, yes, unlike in most places in the world, the heat in Trivandrum, which by sunset is already plenty unbearable, seems to continue to mount for a few hours after the sun goes down, as if spitefully proving that it can.)

Fuming both physically and mentally, I blinked at the darkness and asked myself how I would get through three months of this. Obviously, I considered the fact that this was what it was like to be blind, that for the majority of the people who were living in this building with me, this inability to see anything, this engulfing darkness, this groping around one's own desk to find a book or a glass was the way it was *all the time.*

I sat still and tried to accept the darkness, imagined that I was blind, tried to imagine this darkness as a permanent fact of my life, to believe that this was all I would ever see again. The room seemed to hum and the darkness to press in against me gently from all sides. If I were blind, how would I know day from night? How would I have any sense of time or distance? How would I know anyone? Just at that time I was reading a book called *Touching the Rock,* by a British professor of religion named John Hull who had completely lost his sight in his forties. One sentence in the book had stopped me cold: "It is three years now since I have seen anybody." The thought of being in that position bothered me terribly. Hull had a wife and two children and many colleagues he worked with daily. But three years had passed and he had not *seen* anyone. A paragraph later he wrote, "It distressed me considerably when I realized I was beginning to forget what Marilyn and Imogen [his wife and daughter] looked like." Forgetting the appearance of people you loved was, to my mind, even worse than not seeing anyone. I had said out loud to the book, "God, I would die." And then, a few pages later, Hull wrote, "I find that I am trying to recall old photographs of myself, just to remember what I look like. I discover with a shock that I cannot remember....Is this one of the reasons why I often feel I am a mere spirit, a ghost, a memory?" and it scared me so badly I had to put the book down and focus on something else.

If given the news that I was truly permanently blind, I'm certain that I would become completely hysterical, like the pitiful soldier in *All Quiet on the Western Front*. I, too, would sob and scream pathetically, *I can't see! I can't see!* And then I would become furious and try to fight the blindness somehow, literally pushing at whatever was around me in the belief that if I pushed enough, I'd be able to see again. And when that failed and I had exhausted myself, I would become inconsolable. And then utterly despondent. I would give up fighting and beg for the relief of death.

Being blind was too difficult to imagine, too far beyond my conceptual reach. I tried to relax in the chair, and the more I gave in to the dark, the less the pressure felt like a threat and the more it became like an embrace. I was sweating profusely. I placed my hand on the desk to position myself in relation to something, to anchor myself. By now I was well aware how graceful and efficient, calm and patient the blind were, though they lived in perpetual darkness. I stood up and decided to see how gracefully, patiently, calmly, and efficiently I could put myself to bed in the complete dark.

I did not get terribly far that night before I banged my forehead smartly on the edge of my bunk bed and shouted "Fuck it!" so loudly that my two completely blind neighbors from the room next to mine came running to my screen door to check on me. And how quickly they came running!

One of them, Yoshimi, who was Japanese, said apprehensively, "Rose? Are you all right?"

Embarrassed, I said, "I'm fine, thank you, girls. I just banged my head in the dark."

"Bleeding?" Kyila said. Kyila was from Tibet.

"No, just painful and annoying."

Yoshimi laughed. "I bang my head too."

"And I bang my head also," Kyila said supportively.

"Yes," I said, "but do you lose your temper the way I do when you bang your head?"

Yoshimi said in her nearly flawless English that she could not afford to lose her temper all day long every time she did something clumsy.

Kyila said, "And also we are so used to this."

Their voices were warm and amused and somehow sweetly innocent coming at me out of the night. Their concern was genuine. I said, "We had a power cut. I'm not very good in the dark."

"We know it," Kyila said.

I assured them that I was all right and that they could go back to bed.

"We were not in bed," Yoshimi said.

"You weren't? What were you doing?"

"Reading," Yoshi said.

"Organizing my clothes," Kyila said.

"And so, Rose, if everything is okay, then good night."

I said good night to the girls, and, since I could not read, sort my clothes, or do anything else productive in the dark, I went to bed with my hand wrapped in toilet paper, because I couldn't find the Band-Aids I had brought with me.

I lay in the narrow bed, roasting and unwashed, and realized that when in the village of Nemom Po, one must nightly do as the blind do. One must fumble around one's bedroom, banging one's shins and knocking one's head and spilling water, and while doing it, one must show a blind person's patience, which it occurred to me was akin to an Indian person's patience.

The afternoon before, I was walking in the rain up Mahatma Gandhi Road in Trivandrum at four forty-five when I saw three beautifully dressed women coming out of an office building after a long day of work. They began to make their way up the street when suddenly they spotted a city bus coming toward them, and from the way they reacted at the sight of it, I understood that this was the perfect bus, the one bus that would get them home swiftly and without need of a transfer or a long walk at the end of the line. And what luck to have found it so quickly! They looked profoundly delighted, a delight that electrified their pretty brown faces. They began to run toward the bus stop at the end of the block, waving six arms at the driver to stop him as he drove past, their copper bangles rattling up their forearms to their narrow elbows. They shouted and gestured and smiled eagerly, their white teeth flashing in confidence, as though the driver were a dear old friend. But the driver reached the stop before they did, collected some passengers, and then stepped on the accelerator and roared off just as they arrived, choosing to ignore them as they knocked on the door of the bus.

How did the women react to the frustration and misfortune? They laughed. They laughed at the driver's blunt insensitivity. They stood at the bus stop, shoulders back, spines straight, heads high, laughing at their bad luck as they settled in for the usual hour's wait for the next bus. They exchanged a few light words, smiling and sighing cheerfully in a way that meant it would certainly have been too much to expect this little thing to go their way, that they had gotten ahead of themselves in their ambition to get home quickly, that in fact it was probably much better that they had to wait here in the dirty rain another hour. They patted their sleek hair and stared eagerly up Mahatma Gandhi Road, smiling brightly and with a patience that from my perspective resembled insanity.

I pictured myself under the same circumstances. The image was not pleasant. Had the same thing happened to me, I would have removed my shoe and heaved it at the driver's window as he passed, hoping to smash the glass and hit him on his petty, insensitive head. I would have run after the bus, one foot bare, hurling after it every foul word I could think of. And my entire evening would have been thoroughly poisoned by anger.

I exaggerate. Of course I would not have done exactly that, but I would in my heart have done it. In my heart and mind, I would have condemned the man to a life of suffering and pain, and as we know, it's the thought that counts. Patience is admittedly not my strong point. I often think that I must be the most impatient person I know aside from two of my brothers. (The third brother is patient to a fault; his patience sometimes makes me impatient.) I regret this. I have consciously tried to become a more patient person, but at fifty-one, I still have not come close to the degree of patience I wish for, have not achieved the superior equanimity I hope for, have not managed to tame a shred of my inherent irritability. I was born impatient and annoyed.

I fitted the crook of my elbow over my eyes and thought then about the patience the newly blind would have to cultivate, and eventually I fell asleep knowing that I would never be able to achieve that level of patience. I would never be a well-adjusted blind person. I was not even a well-adjusted sighted person.

I dreamed that night that Sabriye Tenberken was not really blind, that she had only been pretending to be blind. In the dream she reacted with horror to a motorcycle accident we had witnessed, and suddenly I understood not only that she could see perfectly well but that for years she had been conning the world with an elaborate ruse of blindness. In the dream, the revelation was disturbing and impressive. But, of course, it was only a dream. Sabriye was indeed completely blind. The dream was surely an expression of my own wonder at her grace and complete ease with her blindness. The more I got to know her, the more her blindness receded from my consciousness, until it seemed not to be there at all.

A few hours later I was woken by an unpleasant sensation on my skin, a general stinging all over my body, as though the bedsheets had been scattered with fiberglass particles. I threw the top sheet off but the stinging continued. When it became unbearable, I climbed down the ladder from my bunk and tried the light switch, and mercifully the lights came on. I climbed back up and didn't have to look hard at the bed before I realized that it was full of tiny red ants. Hundreds and hundreds of them. I stood on the ladder, staring with disbelief. Then I yanked the sheets off the bed, went out to the balcony—where I heard some living thing of considerable heft skitter away from my bare feet—and shook the sheets over the railing as hard as I could. The night was dense but for a distant light glowing feebly but hopefully in a little house beyond the trees. (Every light in Nemom Po tended to look feeble but hopeful.) An unidentified creature clacked below me on the ground. A bird down toward the lake whooped loudly in long rising notes, as if practicing a tonic scale. I heard what could only have been a coconut thumping heavily to the ground from a great height. I went inside, put the sheets back on the bed, found my flashlight, turned the light off, climbed up, lay down again, stashed the flashlight under my pillow the way people in war zones stash guns, and fell asleep for an hour or so before I was awakened again by the same burning on my skin. I sighed very heavily at the ceiling. Then I fished out my flashlight and shone the light on my legs. The bed was again full of flesh-eating ants. Where the hell were they coming from? I got up, spanked the ants off my body, repeated the sheet-shaking exercise, and climbed wearily and with a great sense of futility back into the untrustworthy bed.

At six in the morning I was awoken by a shockingly shrill noise, like a police whistle being frantically blown in a riot. It was a bird in the mango tree outside my window. I got up, bleary-eyed, and looked around the room. There was a bloodstain on the wall near the bathroom and broken glass on the desk; the inked words in my notebook were dissolved by the water I had spilled, and my cell phone lay squarely in the top right corner of the desk, taunting me. I went into the bathroom to find blood all over the floor, my toothbrush and comb lying in the toilet, and beneath the sink an enormous puddle of ants feasting on spilled cough syrup—the unknown object I had knocked off the sink the night before. Leading directly to the puddle was a long solid line of ants marching boldly into the bathroom through the seam around the small window. I filled a bucket with water and splashed the ants down the shower drain.

I went out onto the balcony and saw, in the thinly dawning light, still more ants rounding the corner of the building in a dense unbroken river that ran the entire length of the outer wall. I traced the river's flow under my screen door, across the bedroom floor, up the leg and framework of the bed, and into the upper bunk. I then began to mutter profanities. With a wet rag I wiped the bed and the floor clean, dropping the rag now and then into a full bucket of water to drown the hundreds of ants that clung to it. Then I brought the bucket out to the balcony and splashed its contents against the outer wall of the building, thereby sweeping a good segment of the marching line of ants to the ground. I repeated the process several times, then went around to the staircase at the front of the building and splashed the ants from the opposite end of the wall until the entire dark line of them was obliterated. Somewhere beneath all that moist underbrush visible from my balcony, another freshly hatched army of ants was already organizing, already stampeding its way toward my room, but I didn't know that then. I didn't know that in the jungle of Kerala these lines of intruding ants were famous, renewable, and unending. I didn't know then that my hydropathic remedy against them would become a daily task (sometimes twice daily), as necessary and natural to me as brushing my teeth and combing my hair.

I took the mop from my bathroom and went out to my balcony again, where an irate chipmunk clinging to a nearby palm tree was screeching demonically. It was six fifteen; already I was sweating, and dizzy with exhaustion.

Muttering rather loudly now, I mopped up the water I had spilled all over the balcony floor, and when I looked up for a moment I saw, through the palm trees and the smoky morning mist, Sabriye Tenberken striding briskly down the dirt road toward the institute. I leaned on my mop and watched her move. She had the look of a person who had already accomplished several hours of work and was raring to accomplish a great deal more. She fairly flew, wielding her cane like a broadsword, daring the jungle with it.

# The Blind Leading
# the Sighted

The first class I taught at the IISE took place at seven in the morning in a bright, clean room in the brand-new classroom building. The walls of the room had been painted butter yellow, and toward their tops was a fanciful dado of stonework. At the center of the room was a long oval table surrounded by chairs. At seven in the morning, it was already hot enough that I had to open the windows wide and switch on the ceiling fan that hung above the table. Through the windows I could see wands of sunlight slanting through the coconut palms and mango trees, teasing the morning mist. Though it was hot, the ground and the shrubbery were still damp with dew. Wherever the sun struck the campus rooftops, wisps of mist danced upward. Standing at the window, I could smell burning coconut husks, the damp earth, the chemical smell of the wax the classroom floors had been polished with, and, faintly, the muddy water of the lake. Cicadas drummed up a metallic background buzz, like a power saw eating its way through an oak plank; the noise was so constant it had a way of eventually receding entirely from one's consciousness and then unexpectedly returning full force at moments of drifting attention. Carrion crows crouched on the roof of the dining room shouting their hysterical protest at some invisible menace. Now and then an unidentifiable insect the size of a hummingbird swayed and lurched against the window screens hard enough to cause a small thumping noise. Two slender Indian women, housekeepers, came out of the office building with buckets and mops and glided up the brick walkway toward the dormitory. The women were dressed in saris so colorful and elegant that they looked nothing like poverty-stricken Nemom Po residents on their way to scrub toilets and everything like diplomats on their way to an embassy cocktail party. Beyond them in a garden bed, a skeletal, barefoot, knobby-kneed old man stood hacking at the damp red earth with a pickax. He was naked but for a strip of rag tied around his waist. Every time he raised the heavy ax over his head, his ribs stood out in shocking relief.

The purpose of this first class was to determine what sort of help the students needed with their basic English. Several of the other students—the South African woman, the Kenyans, the Norwegian woman, Yoshimi the Japanese woman, the Sierra Leonean, the man from Saudi Arabia, and the Ghanaians—were already fluent in English and didn't need this course in English conversation. I would be working with them on other subjects. But the rest of the students had wildly varying degrees of skill in English and needed a great deal of practice.

We sat that morning around the long oval table, eleven students and I. Although I had been on campus with them for four days already, I noticed for the first time how clean and well groomed they were, how polite and prompt. Though they had had only a short time to acquaint themselves with the campus, not a single one out of eleven was late to the class. About half of them arrived with white canes, and some carried Braille styli and boards in order to take notes. Jessie, the German girl, and Khom, the Nepalese man, came into the room at the same time with their white canes and both tried to sit down in the same chair. Victor, the largest of the three Liberian men, came in and tried to sit down on top of me, and when he realized what he had done and understood from the sound of my voice that I was the teacher, he was mortified and backed away and said in his strong, ringing voice, "Oh! Auntie Rose, I am sorry. Please forgive me." The Liberians had immediately begun calling me auntie because, they explained, I was older than they and it would be rude for them to address me simply by my first name. I was older than Victor by a mere five years. Though they knew English well, the Liberians were in the class to work on their pronunciation.

There was a screen door on the classroom, and several of the students who had never encountered such a door before walked directly into it on their way in, banging their noses on it, not realizing it was there because it had so little mass and reported no echo. After walking into it they put out their hands and felt the screen with expressions of surprise, puzzlement, and curiosity. I had to explain to some of them what the screen was for.

I asked the students to introduce themselves one by one. Johnson, sitting to my left, raised his chin and began to speak to the ceiling fan, his brown hands laid flat upon a yellow page of Braille notes on the table in front of him. "I am Johnson K. Kortu, blind, from Liberia," he said. "I am grateful to God that we are counted among the living. My mother is late, but my father is alive. I am thirty-eight years old."

Johnson had a gentle self-containment, an aura of stillness that commanded respect. He had a strong brow, a broad flat nose, thick lips, and an enormous, ready smile. His large head, shaved to near baldness, was impressive—it had the perfect roundness of a cannon-ball. To shade his blind eyes, he wore the huge dark glasses of a rock star. A deep vertical line of a scar appeared at the right side of his forehead, traveled downward in the direction of his right eye, and disappeared behind the dark lenses. There was another smaller scar at his hairline in the center of his forehead. He was dressed in a lime-green suit of lightweight linen; the suit had been so crisply starched and pressed that the creases at the front of his trouser legs were sharp as the folds in a paper airplane.

Like the other two Liberian students, James and Victor, Johnson was a Christian minister and had adopted a preacher's emphatic style of public speaking. Many of his sentences began with "By the good grace of Almighty God," and he addressed the group of listeners as "my people." Often he repeated a simple sentence for dramatic effect, and like his two compatriots', his accent was particularly congested and difficult to understand. All three of them had a habit of dropping consonants, particularly the consonant at the end of a word, leaving the previous vowel dangling. The word *respect* sounded like "respeh," the word *good* was "gooh," *bad* was "bah," *interaction* sounded like "intahasho," and the word *and* was a lonely little "a." Arriving in Trivandrum, the Liberians were impressed to find that India was blessed with electricity. Because of the Liberian civil war, they had not had electricity in their homes for a very long time. They marveled that there was hot water in the dormitory showers, and when Victor—at forty-two the oldest of the three—was introduced to the washing machines in the laundry room, he crouched down and examined one of them very carefully with his hands, praised God once or twice, and asked whether someone could show him (a man who had been washing his clothes by hand for thirty years) how this wonderful machine was to be operated.

On their first day at the institute, the Liberians, who had never flown in an airplane until that week, told me that the most remarkable event of their journey from Monrovia to Trivandrum was their experience of the moving sidewalk in the Dubai airport. Progressing through the airport toward a connecting flight, they had unwittingly walked onto the moving belt, and within seconds all three of them had fallen down in a jumble of carry-on luggage and white canes. "We did not know what had happened to us!" Victor said, laughing. They had never been on an airplane before, but the experience of flying was as nothing compared to that thoroughly unexpected and inexplicable electronic sidewalk.

In class now, Johnson continued, speaking slowly, dragging his words out, pausing between sentences, carefully arranging his thoughts but with no contrivance or self-consciousness. Though his style had studied, preacherly flourishes, it was also humble. He seemed to be reliving his experience as he spoke, and the emotion in his voice, a kind of stunned disbelief, was genuine. "In my country, Liberia, if a child is blind, they want to kill that child because he is a burden." Silence. "What good can come from that child?" Silence. "They teach the blind child nothing. Yes, I tell you! Nothing! They tie a rope to a bush beyond the house and attach the other end to the house. They tell the child, 'When you have to pee, you hold that rope and follow it to the end, pee there behind the bush and follow the rope back straightly.'" Silence. "The child is like an animal, sitting useless all day. All day!"

It would try my patience and yours for me to re-create in print what Johnson's words actually sounded like; I could see from the looks on the faces around the table that quite a few of the students were straining to understand him. Several of them sat with their heads cocked in an effort to hear him better. In addition to his heavy accent, Johnson had a tic of speech that involved the occasional rapid-fire repetition of the conjunction *to* or *and,* as though he had got hung up on the word. It was not a stutter but a kind of temporizing. He would say, "You ah respossah to to to to to to to tick kee da chah" ("You are responsible to take care of the child") or "Come a a a a a a a lah" ("Come and learn"). At moments of extreme incomprehension, I interrupted his monologue and repeated what I thought he had said, and if I was wrong, he corrected me patiently and without offense.

"In 1996," he continued, "I was blinded in Monrovia when a

rocket-propelled grenade exploded against a wall I was standing beside. There was a civil war. Charles Taylor the warlord wanted nothing good for the people, just power for himself." Silence. "Power for *himself!* I had stopped going to school because of the war. There was no support for students. I was selling things in the market in Monrovia to make my living. I was twenty-six when I was blinded. The doctor told me, 'I'm sorry, your sight has been destroyed.'"

At this Johnson raised his hands over the table, fingers spread wide as if to show that that was it, there was not a thing at all that he could do about it. (Only four of us in the room were able to see his hands, and two of us were seeing them very poorly.) I noticed that his sunglasses were too tight for him; their plastic arms made pronounced indentations in the soft flesh at his temples. The brand name written on the sides of the sunglasses was *Ray & Ban.* He dropped his hands into his lap and sat back in his chair. "I felt discouraged. Yes! Discouraged. My friends who used to come around me would not come around me again." He paused and exhaled wearily. "This did cause me to live in a different world—the world of invisibility. My family understood I got blind. Instead of helping me, they tried to send me away to relatives in the rural area. My people, let me tell you." Silence. "I had a biological brother who used to tease me because I was blind. He said, 'Brother, you are blind and there is nothing useful you can do now. You must go to the country.'"

Johnson clasped his hands, fingers intertwined, on the table before him, and for a moment he looked like a handcuffed prisoner. "But I refused to go. I said to my brother, 'If you want me to go to the country, you must force me. You must tie me up and carry me there! Yes! I say, tie me up!'"

The two other Liberians at the end of the table, also wearing very large dark glasses, their faces shining in the morning heat, supported Johnson with murmurings of "Praise God!"

This was more of a personal introduction than I was expecting, but I had no desire to stop it. I was interested in the story and drawn in by Johnson's style, and I could see by the expressions on his classmates' faces that they were too. He went on: "My brother said to me, 'One thing about you, brother Johnson, you have a big mouth!'"

Several of the students laughed at this, and hearing them laugh, Johnson smiled, encouraged. He stated gravely that he had refused to go to the country and so was rejected by his family. He ended up begging for food and money on street corners. Eventually he discovered that there was a school for the blind in Monrovia. He stayed in the city and attended the school, determined to finish the education that had been interrupted. Having completed his education, he began to teach and earn money, and eventually the same brother who had taunted him came to him seeking financial help. Johnson said, "I saw it in my heart to help my brother."

At this, Pynhoi, a tiny, cheerful, heavily bespectacled young woman from northeast India who had been sitting literally on the edge of her seat throughout Johnson's story, suddenly blurted out at the top of her voice, "Oh! Such a strong man that is!"

At the alarming and unexpected sound of Pynhoi's voice, the two Liberians at the far end of the table chimed in in agreement: "Praise God, he is strong!"

Startled by their response, Pynhoi covered her small face with her hand and ducked down in her seat. Then, slowly straightening up, she raised her glasses higher on her nose with the tip of her index finger and strained to see the Liberians with her feeble eyes. She seemed delighted to have elicited a response from these two Africans. She turned to Johnson and said expectantly, "Mr. Jason, you can please continue that tale."

But Johnson seemed to have wound his story down. "That, my people, is my tale until today. I came to International Institute to continue my education so that one day I can help the blind people of Liberia."

"Praise God," Victor said.

Swept up, Pynhoi said, "Praise!"

I thanked Johnson and asked Jessica, sitting beside him, to introduce herself. Jessica was a twenty-six-year-old from Germany. Born prematurely, she had suffered retinopathy, a common problem in premature babies caused by an underdevelopment of blood vessels in the retina and often exacerbated by too much oxygen in the incubator. Jessica was blind by the time she was a few weeks old. Jessica's English vocabulary was good but she had had very little practice speaking. She spoke haltingly and in a monotone, like a child reading aloud, separating each word from the next with a short pause. She was self-deprecating and often made references to how stupid she was, which in fact she was not. Within a week of meeting her, I understood that she was one of the most intelligent and original students at the school.

Now Jessica said, "I am Yessie from Germany and my English is not so well. I am sorry. Where I lived in Germany, blind children were not allowed to go to normal kindergarten. I was sent to a boarding school when I was three years. They beat me. My parents both were working. My father was an engineer on the sea, driving boats. My mother worked in a bank."

Jessica went on to say that eventually she was integrated into a regular school, where she had to work harder than the other students because she was blind. The other students didn't want to mingle with her because of her blindness. And because she was the only blind student, she was treated as special. "For me it was a big problem to have this special position," she said. "I did not want to be special or different. I wanted to be normal, like everyone else. I have made a really good examination at that school. I was the best in the class, but I did not want to be the best. Sometimes I wanted to be lazy and be like the other students and have fun. I am a little bit juvenile and I am like a child and I want to relax."

Jessica's hair was the exact pale yellow-blond of corn silk and was cut in a jagged shag around her face. Her face was pale and long and narrow, and her eyes had a slightly Asian slant. Her left eye wandered freely as she talked. She was thin, with long arms and legs, and she had already taken to going shoeless around the campus. As she spoke she dangled her hands limply above the table, like the paws of a begging dog, and stirred them in the air in small explanatory circles. Jessica's personality—her frankness, good humor, and unpredictability—made her entirely appealing. There was a refreshing mood of insubordination about her. She had a habit of grinning, ducking her head, and raising her shoulders as if in self-defense whenever she tossed out some provocative or witty line.

"Most disabled persons in Germany are unemployment," she said. "It's because of many people's opinion that the disabled people can't live independent life and can't work accurately. They think we are retarded." She grimaced and made a moronic lowing sound to illustrate for us the essence of abject mental retardedness, then she laughed with her white fingers to her mouth. "Am I like this? No! I think it is very important that people change their attitudes about disabled people. You know what I mean? They have to have more understandment about the blind and disabled. It is trickical for a blind person to express to a sighted person how she can live alone and take care of herself. So, my English is not very well. You will think, *Oh, so stupid girl that is! Maybe she really is retarded.* I am sorry my English is not better. Okay, and that is my introduction."

When she had finished talking Jessie dropped her hands into her lap and lowered her head until her chin was resting on her chest, and suddenly she appeared to have passed out. The breeze from the ceiling fan made the fine hair on her head twitch. When I thanked her for telling us about herself, she did not raise her head but lifted a hand in the air and rotated it from the wrist in a signaling way, as if to say, *It*

*was my pleasure, and I am actually not unconscious. I am still with you.*
*Carry on.*

Next it was Pynhoi's turn. On being asked to speak, Pynhoi slid farther forward in her seat until she hardly seemed to be sitting on it at
all. "Pynhoi Tang. That is my name. And really I am coming from a
small village in Shillong Province, north and east part of India. And
okay, so I am twenty-three years old."

She did not look twenty-three. She looked fourteen. She had the
body of a child and she dressed in the utilitarian cotton trousers and
collared shirt of a Catholic schoolboy. Her name was pronounced
"Pin-hoy." She spoke without pause or punctuation—the rapid-fire
clatter of a sewing machine. The night before, she told me that when
she was very young her family had been nomads, constantly moving
and sleeping in a bamboo hut with a grass roof. Wherever they went
they simply threw a new hut together and moved in. They survived
by eating whatever animals her father could catch and kill with a bow
and arrow, a spear, or, sometimes, with his bare hands. Cheerfully she
rattled off for me the various types of animals she had eaten in her life:
tiger; monkey; wild pig; squirrel; rat; some sort of forest rat that she
could not specifically define except to say that it had a large nose; deer;
horse; snakes of many kinds; dog; cat; frog; forest hen (also not precisely definable); turtle; lizard; rabbit; this; that; another thing; crow,
turkey, sparrow, parakeet, and really any bird at all except eagle. When
I asked why they didn't eat eagle, she said, "Because we doon ting dat
bahd is healty."

Pynhoi went about with an expectant, ever-present smile on her
face, as if constantly prepared to be surprised and entertained. Her
pale brown skin was smooth as a toddler's but for a small dark mole
on her left cheek. She wore her hair in a ponytail that swept down her
back. "And okay so I had lot of trouble with my eyes, my seeing was
not good since I was young, and I had one teacher who help me in

school but after grade six no one help me so I stop school. My parents were poor. And teachers not patient and that is the problem with them. They must respect what life we have, but there is too many in the villages who don't get help because of disability. So, there comes my mind thinking, *What about the others who don't get help?* Some of the parents, it seem they don't like their children because they are disability. And when I finish my study I want to help the disability, and I never dream that I would go so far from my home place and come to here in Vellayani. And I am so happy to meet all you new my friends coming from the far places of the world."

Pynhoi laid her arms flat on the table and peered around the room at her new friends, beaming gamely behind the dense lenses of her glasses. She seemed hardly able to believe her good fortune. "Oh, I am *so* happy," she said with irrepressible sincerity and appreciation.

I thought Pynhoi was finished and moved to invite Gompo Gyentzen to speak. But Pynhoi was not finished. She went on, telling us that when she got a bit older she went to an integrated boarding school with sighted students and that occasionally the sighted students used to test her strength and mind because she was blind. "It was difficult," Pynhoi said. "I had to show that I was able to do things. I had a friend, she want to cook something, so she just took the basin from me. I told her don't do this for me. This is not your, it is mine, and she beat me, and the next day when she went to beat me again, I just hold her and squeeze her there." One day when the sighted students were playing basketball, Pynhoi asked to play with them. They told her she couldn't play because she couldn't see. "I said, 'Let me see if I can play.' But they pull me down and trap me. And they said, 'How can she go to college, she is totally blind!' "

Pynhoi peered vaguely around the room, not smiling now. Again I thought she was finished, and I began to speak. But, no, she was not yet finished.

"Not only I finish college but I come here to Trivandrum. When I came traveling to Trivandrum last week I am in the airport and I try to make a phone call in the airport but I had no coins so I beg one rupee off of each person I meet in the airport and my friend who came to say good-bye to me tell me, 'Pynhoi, by time you arrive at Trivandrum, you will be a blind beggar!'"

She tittered at the notion. "So I find enough rupees to make the phone call. Then, while I am talking on phone, the airline man at the gate is waving to me to come along, my plane is leaving, but I cannot to see well enough him, then finally he come to me and grab my arm and pull me and because I think he is kidnap me I shout—"

She gripped the edge of the table to brace her little body and demonstrated for us exactly the piercing way in which she shouted *Help! Help!* at the top of her lungs. All the chins around the oval table lifted a little higher at the shocking sound. At the punch line of her own story, Pynhoi began to laugh so hard she doubled over and gasped for breath, and the sound of her tee-hee-ing and snorting and gasping was so amusing and infecting that the others began to laugh too. Pynhoi had worked herself up into a frenzy with her rambling monologue. She was helpless with laughter. She had to hold on to her glasses to keep them from falling off her face. Tears of mirth streamed down her little round cheeks. She had started to tell us a little about herself and before we knew it, she had thrown in the basin and the basketball and the kidnapping too. This, we would soon come to learn, was her habit. Once Pynhoi began to talk, she picked up speed and found it difficult to stop. She talked so much and so fast and veered off on so many tangents that it was easy to fade out while she was talking, not unlike the natural human response to the thrum of the cicadas, and yet often when you faded back in you realized with a start that what she was saying had great logic to it, a moral, a worthy punch line, or simply something very poignant. Her rambling had a touching coherence.

Above all, Pynhoi had the gift of being able to laugh at herself. She said now, "Okay and now I am talk so much, oh my God," and sat back in her chair, clearly resolved to keep quiet. But she could not quite do it; she was compelled to add one more thing. "And my maddah sometime scold me for my loud voice. She say, 'Doddah, your voice so loud and sharp it is like a sword! It can cut down a tree with one chop!'"

Her classmates laughed, and Jessie lifted her head from her chest to tell Pynhoi, "Yah, Pynhoi, so I think your mother is right!"

Pynhoi grinned and sank lower in her seat.

Gyentzen, sitting beside Pynhoi, was the thinnest person I had ever seen walking upright, thinner even than the Indian gardener outside the building. He was so thin that he could wear a wristwatch strapped above his elbow. Beneath his cotton T-shirt, his shoulders looked like the wings of a wooden coat hanger. He had a large face with a strong jaw and pronounced cheekbones, a handsome Tibetan icon of a face. Gyentzen was shy and quiet and completely blind. His eyes were shrouded behind a dense white film, and his thick dark hair, cut short, was like a glossy fur hat upon his head. That morning he sat holding hands with Kyila, who was sitting beside him. He and Kyila had attended Sabriye's Braille Without Borders school in Lhasa and had essentially grown up together. They were not lovers, nor were they siblings. They simply had a habit of holding hands or linking arms, as blind acquaintances often do.

I had met Gyentzen once before in Tibet and I mentioned that now to the class. I asked Gyentzen to tell us something about himself. He smiled and lowered his head and moved closer to Kyila until their shoulders were touching. He remained silent, grinning into his lap. Finally he said, "My name is Gompo Gyentzen. You can say Gyentzen. And…" He made a fist of his right hand and dropped it five or six times into his left palm. "And my name means 'victory.'"

Kyila, whose blind eyes were perpetually crossed, leaned slightly away from Gyentzen to listen to him.

"I come from Tibet," he said. "And"—his fist fell into his left palm again, an expression of apprehensiveness—"and twenty-two years old." He paused, visibly searching for the next word. "Now I am in India." He paused again, let out a dry laugh of surrender, laid his bony forearms on the table, lowered his chin onto them, closed his damaged eyes, pressed his lips together, and stopped talking completely. The sudden silence allowed the whine of the cicadas and the vomiting of the crows to fill up the room.

Kyila tilted closer to Gyentzen now, her mouth hanging open, her oval face utterly frozen, waiting with the cocked and concentrated appall of a woman crouched behind her bedroom door listening to the sounds of the burglar downstairs. She waited in vain, for nothing else was forthcoming from Gyentzen. The silence went on long enough that finally Kyila gave him a gentle nudge with her elbow; their friendship was so intimate that clearly she felt a personal responsibility for his performance. Gyentzen sat up and whispered something furtive to her in Tibetan; she whispered back with a look of disbelief on her face.

I asked Gyentzen if he was finished. He dropped his fist onto his thigh in frustration and chagrin, sighed through his teeth. "Finish."

Gyentzen obviously spoke English poorly, and having to perform in front of ten colleagues had paralyzed him. Kyila's face was clouded with disappointment. Since I already knew something about him and had read the introductory essay that accompanied his application to the institute, I asked his permission to tell the class a bit more about him. He was relieved. "Okay, yes."

Gyentzen had lost his sight at age nine and was told that the cause of his blindness was bad karma and therefore he would not be able to do anything with his life. His parents were farmers. By chance he met Paul and Sabriye when he was twelve. At Braille Without Borders he learned Tibetan, Chinese, mathematics, computer technology, and Braille. After graduating from BWB he attended a regular school with three other blind students; they were the first blind children ever to be integrated into a mainstream school in Tibet. Upon finishing regular school, he took a job at BWB teaching and printing Braille books for the students. He won a scholarship to study for a month in Thailand, and he and Kyila had gone on a very difficult climbing expedition in the Himalayas with an American climbing team, Paul and Sabriye, and some of the other blind students from Braille Without Borders. An American production company had filmed the expedition and made a documentary about it called *Blindsight*. At one surprising, highly entertaining point in the film, Gyentzen had sung an absolutely raucous Tibetan folk song at the top of his voice.

Kyila giggled, remembering this, and whispered to Gyentzen again. When Gyentzen comprehended what I had just said about his song, his face ignited in a glowing confusion of delight and embarrassment.

"And finally," I said, "I believe Gyentzen's dream is to establish a Braille publishing house and Braille library in Lhasa. Is that correct, Gyentzen?"

He nodded his head and ventured, "That is correct."

"Okay, then, Kyila, would you like to tell us something about yourself?"

Kyila Tsering was a slight, ponytailed young woman in jeans and a T-shirt. She was the one in Lhasa who had passed me in a hallway of the BWB school and determined who I was solely by the way I smelled. Kyila was now twenty-four. She had been born near Mount Everest in a village of eight hundred people. "My father, me, and my train brothers are all blind," she began.

I interrupted her. "Sorry, your *what* brothers?"

"Train."

"I don't know what that means."

"Trains. Two brothers born at the same time."

"You mean *twins?*"

"Yah. Trains."

I asked Kyila to say *twenty.* She said, "Trenty." I asked her to say *twinkling.* "Trinkling." She couldn't pronounce the letter *w,* nor did she know what the letter *w* looked like. Jessie raised her head to confess that she, too, did not know the shape of a *w.* James, one of the Liberians at the end of the table, said, "Me too. I don't know how the double-u looks."

"Okay," I said, "we can work on all that later. Please continue."

"Okay," Kyila said. "So, because we were blind, my mother had to take care of us. I could not go out and play with other children and was not let to do anything for myself. When I first went to Braille Without Borders I was twelve. I didn't know how to dress or wash myself already. I had no education."

At BWB Kyila was delighted to meet other blind students who had had the same experience she had. When she heard that Sabriye, the woman who started the school, was blind, she didn't believe it at first. "I always thought that blind people couldn't do anything except eat and sleep."

After her studies at BWB, Kyila trained to become a professional masseuse. She learned Chinese massage, acupuncture, and physiotherapy. She and a blind friend started their own physiotherapy clinic in Lhasa, and in 2005 she went to England to study English for a year. Her dream was to set up a kindergarten for blind children in Lhasa.

I asked Victor, the oldest Liberian, to introduce himself. He cleared his throat and raised his hands, as if speaking to a congregation from an elevated pulpit. "Good morning, my colleagues. My visionary colleagues, good morning. I am Victor N. G. Gaigai from Liberia, West Africa, and born 1966 unto the blessed union of Mr. and Mrs. Gaigai, who have graciously given birth to fourteen children."

Victor's speech was slow and clearer than Johnson's, but still he had the extremely complicated Liberian accent. He was a big man with the physique of a polar bear: sloping shoulders, a round stomach, and big, solid legs. He walked like an erect polar bear too—flat-footed and tilting side to side, with his big hands swinging. His hair was so short it was like a dark bathing cap on his head. Victor was sweet and gentle, with a polite and ingenuous air, and his hair came to a kind of crest at its top, like a continental divide. He placed his Braille notepad in front of him. "I am a Christian and a family man," he said. "I have four children. I have been working for the blind in the past ten years at the Christian Association of the Blind."

Victor explained that as an infant, he had had the measles, and his eyesight was severely damaged because of it. His parents knew nothing about the disease, and whatever treatment they had given him was not appropriate. At the age of nine he got another eye disease. "One morning, I got up from bed with my eyes swollen up and water running down from them. It was a terrible moment in my life. The sickness forced both eyes out of my head and they were hanging on my cheeks for a whole month."

Not quite believing what I was hearing, I winced, and then, in an attempt at decorum, I tried not to wince, then realized it didn't matter if I made a horrified face, because nobody but Martin Niry of Madagascar, one of the two fully sighted students at the institute, could see my face that clearly. And Martin too was wincing. And so, in fact, was everyone else. I felt I should say something sympathetic, but Victor was intent on his story.

"Within that time my grandmother died, and I could not cry because of my condition. When my grandaunt came to her sister's funeral, she met me in agony. She was frustrated and got angry with my parents: Why they could not have sent for her to prevent this?" The grandaunt went into the bush, collected some chalk, mixed it with herbs, rubbed it on Victor's eyelashes, and soon enough his eyes began to recede back into their sockets. "When they went in," he said, "they twisted in the sockets and I could not see with my right eye, while the left eye vision was very low."

This was like something from the darkest of the Grimms' fairy tales. Martin and I were now grimacing freely at each other. I couldn't see Victor's eyes behind his big sunglasses and was extremely curious to know what they looked like now, some thirty years after all that violent upheaval. Victor said dramatically, "After the incident, my future was very bleak! I was the only blind child in the whole town. I could not go to school because there was no blind school in the district."

When Victor was sixteen, his brother found a grade school for the blind in Monrovia and brought him there. The principal of the school, who was also blind, began to examine Victor with his hands and finally announced that Victor was too tall and too old to attend the school. Nevertheless, he found it in his heart to give Victor a chance. Victor said, "He said he would give me a six months' grace period to learn and complete the entire Braille course to read and write, or else he would give me NTR: Never to Return."

Victor was placed in the beginners' class. I pictured him sitting enormously among the seven-year-old children in the first grade, his big arms slung across a tiny desk. "My colleagues," Victor said, "the first time I saw Braille I almost gave up because I could not recognize anything. However, I decided to take the challenge to learn."

Within six months Victor completed the entire Braille reading and writing course. He was tested by the principal, passed, and was promoted to the second grade. His promotions to the next grades came quickly, one after the next, and after three years he was integrated into a regular school. Not long after he entered this school, the Liberian civil war began, and his education came to an end. "I did not go to school for nine consecutive years," he said. "Instead, I was in our village all those years doing nothing to improve my life."

Images I had seen from the Liberian civil war passed through my mind. Young boys who had been ordered to take hallucinogens, forced to dress in wedding gowns, and then given machine guns and sent to shoot their parents, part of their initiation into the rebel forces. Images of severed heads, shallow graves, legless children, smashed buildings, charred and grotesquely mutilated bodies.

I thanked Victor and asked James to tell us something about himself. James, sitting next to Victor, smiled and adjusted his enormous sunglasses; the lenses of the glasses were besmirched with thumbprints and greasy streaks. He was a handsome man with even features and a stunning smile that blossomed easily and often. He was dressed that morning in a spotless white dashiki with colorful embroidery sewn around its open collar. "I am James Patrick Johnson, Liberian," he said. "My brothers and sisters, let me thank God, who granted us traveling mercy for our journeys to this place. I am forty-one years old. Now, James Patrick Johnson, who is he? He was born unto the blessed union of Mr. Jacob Johnson and Wilkie Johnson, may their souls rest in peace."

James's parents had been poor farmers. Like Victor, he had lost his sight because of measles. "When I was small," he said, "I began to see things upside down. When I said this to people, they thought that I was possessed by demons."

Johnson interrupted James to say, "True! In Liberia, whenever people see a blind person going about his house, they say, 'Now, this man before me must be dealing in witchcraft. He cannot see, but he moves like a man who sees, finding everything and not bumping into something. So! That is witchcraft. Or it is voodoo!'"

James said in agreement, "They say it is voodoo. And this is why people are afraid to cheat you, if you are blind. They think that you will put a curse on them!"

"The truth!" Victor said. "And sometimes they are afraid to mix a blind man's money among their own money. So, the driver of a taxi, he refuse to take your money sometime if you are blind. It make you feel bad."

"It make you feel very bad, I tell you!" Johnson said.

"Brothers!" James said in a rallying way. "This is Lahbeeya! Lahbeeya, oldest country in Africa," and he went on with his life story. One day, American missionaries who had started a school for the blind in his tribal area found little blind James playing in a coconut plantation. They took him home to his parents and asked if he could attend their school. At the school he learned Braille. Subsequently he studied at the Liberian National School for the Blind, and then he entered a regular high school, where he was the only blind student. He grinned mischievously. "One thing. Because I was blind I had the benefit to use a typewriter to make my notes, and because the girls in my class liked the typewriter, they always sat close to me!" By the time James completed high school, the civil war had "ruined the entire country."

"War has set my country back by fifty years," he said. James was, at that point, a teacher at the Liberian National Resource Institute for the Blind. He was married and had three children and his dream was to open a computer institute for the blind in Liberia. "When people have some negative feeling about you, you have to do something to change this. When we applied to this IISE, there was a colleague who was supposed to be sending our e-mails to Paul and Sabriye for us. But he did not send our e-mails, because he was jealous that we wanted this opportunity. I thought he had sent them, but he had not. When we learned this, we became so red! But now, thankfully, I am very, very happy to be counted among the participants here at International Institute," he said, "and thank you very much."

Sitting beside James was Khom Raj Sharma, a twenty-six-year-old from Nepal. No matter the time of day, Khom always resembled a beleaguered stockbroker just home from a long day's work. He wore a dress shirt open at the throat, its sleeves rolled up on his hairy forearms. Two days' worth of beard growth covered the lower half of his face in black velour. His left eye was permanently shut, and all that was visible of the right eye was a sliver of white between its slightly parted lids. Khom had a slow, grave manner and a powerful political conscience. He said in a thick Nepalese accent, "I am Khom Raj Sharma and I am born in 1983 in Nepal. My wife is partially sighted, and we have a baby born six months ago."

Khom had been completely blind in his left eye from the time he was born, and he lost all vision in his right eye when he was eleven years old. "My village was remote," he said, "and my family is very poor. There was no one in my family literate before me, so my parents did not know anything about treating my eyes, so I was forced to become blind. If I tried to write something, I would begin at the top of the paper and, because I could not see, the words would fast be falling down to the bottom of the paper. People ridiculed me. And they laughed at me when I was walking on the street because I couldn't see; they didn't understand that I was blind. I always said that one day I will contribute to society, even though I am blind."

Khom went on to say that he studied Braille, and, after meeting people at the Nepal Association of the Blind, he was inspired to advocate for the rights of the blind and disabled. He was disturbed to find that there existed no library for the blind in all of Nepal, which meant that there were no texts available for the education of blind students beyond grade school. He had traveled to the eastern part of Nepal to teach Braille to blind children. After much searching, he found a Dutch NGO to support his digital library project.

Khom said essentially the same thing his classmates had said about the negative perceptions of the blind in his society: the Nepalese people did not believe that blind people were capable of anything. His goal was to establish a training center for the blind and visually impaired in Nepal to help them become independent. He also wanted to run for office. "Advocacy and unity are needed to put pressure on the Nepalese government to make human-rights policies for the blind and other disabled people," he said. "So, I am lucky to be here with you to improve my knowledge and my skills."

Holiniaina Rakotoarisoa was next. She was a very pretty young woman from Madagascar, with a gentle, conservative manner, naturally arched black eyebrows, and pale brown skin. Her eyes were the opposite of crossed—her left eye veered toward the left, her right eye steered slightly to the right. That morning Holi was wearing a pink T-shirt that said MADAGASCAR across its front. She told us her story in a French-African accent, pausing now and then to find a word. When she was seven years old, she got a disease that affected her eyes, and because she and her family lived in the countryside, there was no physician to help her. She became completely blind.

I looked around the room. So many of these people had lost their eyesight because they lived in rural areas, had no money, and so could get no medical help. Much of the blindness here could probably have been prevented easily under different circumstances.

Holi leaned forward over the table. "After my parents found a doctor in a town, my sight improved a little bit and now I have some vision. I went to join the blind school in Antsirabe. It was the only primary school for blind kids in Madagascar. After that school, I was integrated into the ordinary school with sighted pupils. At that time I had difficulty in my study, because some teachers did not accept to receive a blind person to study in their school. This is why a lot of blind people become beggars. They can get no education."

Holi had had difficulty getting the study aids she needed to keep up in a class of sighted people. At university, her teacher would not allow her to use her Braille typewriter to take notes because the noise of it disturbed the other students. She was forced to spend what little money she had on a tape recorder, cassettes, and batteries. Because many of the books and documents for her courses were not available in Braille, she needed someone to accompany her to the library and read them aloud for her. "Sometimes, if my friends were not available, I had to pay someone else to read for me. It was costing me a lot of money to study."

Holi stopped there and looked at her hands. From watching Holi walk and seeing how she came up to me when she wanted to ask me something, I knew that her vision was minimal. There was caution in the way she approached a door, a painstaking slowness in the way she located an object on a table.

"Sometimes I feel sad when I have difficulty in my life," Holi said. "But I am proud of myself when I am successful. We have in my country humans' rights. But the rights for disabled people has not come yet. I have decided to make a project for the visually impaired people in my country and help them so they will not be dependent on their families. And so that is my story."

Sitting beside Holi was Martin Niry, also from Madagascar. Martin was a fully sighted man of thirty. He was thin, shy, and boyish-looking, with a serious face, a patient, observant air, and a heavy French-Malagasy accent. He explained to us that he had worked for ten years as an educator for the blind and also in Braille book production. He had taken training courses in blind education in South Africa and Tanzania, and his goal was to work in management of social organizations geared toward services for the blind. He was married and had a young son. "It is not easy to discuss education for the blind in a place like Madagascar," he said. "The education of disabled kids is not really supported by the government. It's mostly private associations and foreign NGOs that take a responsibility for them. The best thing I can do is to encourage Malagasy people to think differently about these issues. And that is why I came here to work with all of you and learn better skills. And thank you for giving me a place here."

The last student to introduce himself was Marco, the only student from South America. Marco was forty years old, extremely intelligent and hardworking. Like Khom, Marco had a calm, mature manner and strong political feeling. He was short but had the powerful chest and shoulders of a welterweight boxer. His large face was pale and square, and his eyes were hidden behind square dark glasses that resembled the protective eyewear worn in a chemical laboratory. Marco had a notable underbite and such pronounced eyeteeth that when he smiled, he slightly resembled an English bulldog. His hair was similar to Gyentzen's—dark black, extremely thick, and cut short so that the natural grain of its growth was visible, not unlike a bear's pelt. I had already discovered that although Marco's speech was slow, he had an obsessive passion for the English language and had acquired an impressive English vocabulary. He was in the habit of using words like *querulous* and *banish, ameliorate* and *importune*. Most of what he knew he had learned from the Voice of America and BBC radio. He never let an unfamiliar word go by without asking what it meant or looking it up in his dictionary.

"I am Marco Tulio Benavides," he said. "I am from Colombia. I am married and have one teenage son. I was born blind and my sister was also. My parents, who were illiterate and poor, thought there was no hope for us, and so they went to church and made a Mass with the prayer that my sister and I would die."

To make a Mass means to request, often with a donation of a sum of money, that a priest will celebrate the Mass with a particular intention in mind. I could not imagine that any priest, no matter how corrupt, would be willing to wish death upon a pair of infants and concluded that Marco must have meant that his parents had expressed this prayer in their own hearts.

When Marco was seven years old, his aunt declared that she would take the boy and try to find a cure for his blindness. No cure was found. The aunt encouraged him to study at an institute for the blind, which he did, and when his studies were completed, he returned to his parents' home. "Though we had no money, and there was a lot of discrimination against me," he said, "I was the first blind student to attend and successfully complete the regular primary school education in my town. After a long struggle I got accepted in a regular secondary school."

Marco's classmates at the regular school mocked and taunted him because of his blindness, and their parents complained to the school administration that a disabled child should not be sharing classes with their normal children. "I had difficulties in socializing and getting friends," Marco said, "so most of the time I was alone in the school yard at break time."

Gradually, people realized what a good student Marco was, and they began to change their opinions about him. But good student or no, when he finished school and applied for jobs, he was rejected everywhere because of his blindness. He ended up washing plastic bottles and selling raffle tickets on the street in order to make enough money to support his wife and son. Eventually he was hired as a part-time teacher of the blind, and he and some other blind adults formed an organization in aid of local blind people. "We managed to get funding to provide educational materials for the blind—Braille paper, Braille slates, white canes, tape recorders, cassettes, radios, and other useful things. But still, there is so much more we need to accomplish in my country. And so I am here, like the rest of you, to learn how to continue this work more efficiently."

With ten minutes remaining to our class and the Kerala sun lifting over the palm trees and screwing its vise tighter on the world, I decided to correct some of the mistakes that had been made in the past forty minutes. I looked around the room at the faces. Sweat was beading on the foreheads of some of the men and on the upper lips of some of the women. The armpits of Khom's white shirt were damp. The ceiling fan didn't offer much relief, just stirred the hot air onto our heads. I told Jessica that in English there was no such word as *understandment* or *trickical* (though I quite liked that one) and asked who knew what the correct words were. Marco raised his hand. "Understanding and tricky."

"Right. And also, Jessie, *unemployment* is a noun and therefore people who do not have jobs cannot *be* unemployment. Who knows the correct adjective?"

Marco said, "Unemployed."

"And, Pynhoi," I said, "*disability* is also a noun. People who have a disability are described with what adjective? Who *except* Marco knows it?"

"Crippled!" James blurted.

I couldn't help laughing. "Well, yes, you could say that, but the word *crippled* has negative connotations. Would you refer to yourself as a cripple, James?"

"Never!"

Holi said, "Disabled."

"Right," I said. "And, Gyentzen, Holi used the word *available* earlier. Do you know what that means?"

Marco began to speak, but I cut him short, told him that I knew he knew the answer but that the question was directed to Gyentzen. Marco smiled in acknowledgment; he knew he was a walking English dictionary.

"Gyentzen?" I said.

Gyentzen began with the fist in the palm again.

"If you don't know what a word means—and I'm speaking to all of you and not just to Gyentzen—do *not* let the word go by without asking what it means. This is why you're here. And, Gyentzen, tell me something: Back in Lhasa, were you also a carpenter?"

Gyentzen thought. "Carpenter?"

"A man who makes things out of wood."

He looked properly puzzled. "No."

"I ask this because you are constantly hammering with your right hand."

Martin, who was Gyentzen's roommate, laughed loudly in recognition.

"Do you know what *hammering* is, Gyentzen?" I said.

"No."

"Kyila, please tell Gyentzen what *hammering* is."

Kyila did as I asked, and Gyentzen nearly choked on his own laughter.

Because I wanted Kyila to practice pronouncing the letter *w,* I turned then to the word *twinkling.* Only two people in the class knew what it meant. Unimaginatively I used the example of the stars, and of course that fell flat, for most of the students had never seen the stars or else had seen them so long ago that they couldn't really remember them. Only Johnson, who was blinded late, and Martin, who was not blind at all, knew what I meant. How to explain to a group of blind people what *twinkling* is or how a *w* is shaped? I thought what an odd English class this would be, and I was not quite sure I was prepared to teach it. I said that the quality of twinkling light was a bit like the feel of raindrops on one's arm. I got out of my chair and lightly drummed my fingertips on the back of the hand of each person who didn't know the word and tried to attach the sensation to the flickering, pulsating, intermittent quality of a twinkling light. But then, of course, I had to back up and explain what light was like for those few who had no knowledge of it.*

---

*Most blind people who can be said to have no useful sight are not profoundly blind in the strictest medical sense. Profound blindness describes a completely nonfunctioning retina that has no sensitivity to light whatsoever. Many blind people can see some light in a sensation similar to what you might experience if you lay in the sun and closed your eyes. Your eyes are closed, yet still you see light, and even a color that occupies the spectrum between yellow and red, and if, while lying there, you pass your hand close before your face, your eyes, though closed, will register your hand's shadow. You cannot truly see, yet your retina continues to function.

How to describe light? It was like trying to define life after death or the origin of the universe. I labored to compare the effect of light on the eyes to the effect of heat on one's skin or strong taste—a wedge of lemon, say—on one's tongue. I attempted to compare it to a strong smell—mint, cigarette smoke, chlorine. Finally, a few of them said, "I think I understand."

Throughout this exercise I was reminded of something I had read: A blind woman who had regained her sight insisted, "You can't tell a person how anything looks unless he has once had eyes that saw. The words don't mean a thing to him." Perhaps blind people didn't understand, but they often used the language of the sighted, and I thought that to know roughly what a person meant when he said *twinkling* might be useful to them one day.

Although it wasn't really necessary for blind people to know the shapes that made up the Roman alphabet, I wanted to convey to them what a *w* looked like. I asked the students to put the three middle fingers of their left hands flat on the edge of the table and then spread those fingers as wide as possible. Then I told them to trace the outline of those fingers with the index finger of the right hand. They did this, and several of them said, "Ah!" When I announced that the class had come to an end, some of the students reached for their white canes that lay folded on the floor at their feet,[*] and they all stood and began to make their way out the door. A few of them walked into the chairs that had not been pushed back to the table; several of them collided near the door, and Victor walked himself into the wrong corner and had to work around the periphery of the room with the tip of his cane tapping low against the walls until he felt the screen door. This was

---

*Most modern white canes are constructed of three or four lengths of hollow aluminum tubing held together by an elastic cord inside, which allows the cane to be folded to a compact size, very like the ribs of a camping tent.

only the second or third time they had been in this building, and some went out the door and turned the wrong way down the hall. I followed them out and redirected them. At the end of the hallway, near the entrance to the building, a few began to stumble up the staircase to the second floor, laughed at the mistake, corrected themselves, and finally found the exit.

I watched them leave the building and head off down the footpath at the center of the campus. None of them walked in a way that suggested fear, though the campus was still unfamiliar to them. I marveled again at the patience they exuded and the trust they placed in the physical world, qualities that I once would have described as desperate necessity but now perceived as confidence and self-possession. This sense of ease seemed to broadcast a fundamental connection to the world that was, I suspected, deeper and more elementary than the one I had.

# Perception

Days at the IISE passed with a regular, unwavering rhythm. Breakfast at six thirty; classes at seven; a general assembly in the auditorium with group discussions, presentations, and speeches by teachers and students alike; more classes; lunch; a break in the hottest hours of the afternoon; a class again in the evening; dinner at six thirty; staff meetings; and then a half-hour power cut. As the days went by, without noticing it, I became used to living among the blind. I became used to the sound of white canes scraping and tapping down the walkway outside my bedroom door, to the clacking sound the folded canes made as the students shook them back to their upright positions at the end of a class. I grew used to the sound of heads knocking against the frame of my bedroom window (it opened outward, like a door, and the wind occasionally pushed it into the path of students hurrying down the walkway). I grew used to the sight of a hundred horizontal finger streaks on the dormitory windows from all the hands that reached out to feel their way along the corridor. I got used to the shocking gunshot sounds of screen doors slamming and to shouting, "Quit letting those screen doors slam! I thought you blind people didn't like loud noises." I got used to the laughter and the hoots I received in response to that comment. I got used to people walking into me, goosing me and tripping me with their white canes, sitting down on top of me, accidentally taking my plate, my fork, my water glass at meals. At the dinner table, I got used to ducking full cups of hot tea that I regularly saw (usually at the last moment from the corner of my eye) barreling toward my head in the hands of passing students. (A good number of people ended up with brown stains down the backs of their shirts as a result of these dining room accidents.) I got into the habit of stating to all present that I was leaving the dinner table or leaving a room so that they would not try to talk to me in my absence. (Sabriye had told me that once, when she was sitting in a restaurant in Germany with her father, she had gotten into a heated political argument with him. At some point her father went to the men's room without telling her, and she continued to rant loudly and for an extended period to an empty table.) I learned to guide blind companions on a walk using my voice instead of my arm. I got used to the sight of scarred shins and bruised knees, got used to walking past a completely dark room and hearing many voices coming out of it.

I was, in fact, surprised at how little difference there was between living among the sighted and living among the blind. Blind people at the institute got out of bed in the morning and put on their clothes, went to the dining room, fed themselves, put salt and pepper on their food, made their own toast, ate with forks and knives (except for the few Africans who were in the habit of eating with their hands); after the evening meal, they took turns washing the dishes. They arrived at class on time. They did not have constant accidents or frequently lose their possessions. Nobody fell off a balcony, got electrocuted, caused the school to go up in flames. Nobody drowned while swimming in the lake. Nobody got lost on expeditions into the city. And nobody ever used blindness as an excuse for anything. Nobody ever even referred to his or her own blindness except in a political or sociological context. They were not preoccupied with their blindness. It was just a fact of life.

After countless failed attempts to explain various visual phenomena with examples that would have had meaning only for a sighted person, and after countless failed attempts to use my hands to describe objects and shapes when my hands were invisible to my students, I gradually got used to a much more physical approach to them. Before long I found myself making my points by tapping on their foreheads, holding their heads in my hands, covering their ears, making them trace designs on the table, making them feel shapes that I made with my fingers. I became used to (though never truly adept at) having to describe snow and lightning, steam and fireflies and the moon and a hundred other common sights that they could neither see nor entirely imagine. And I stopped believing that I could ever really hide myself or anything else from them.

At the beginning of the year, before the entire campus was equipped with wireless Internet, there was only one room in which the Internet was available. Students would bring their laptop computers to this room and send and receive e-mails from there. One afternoon I was sitting in the Internet room alone, typing a long e-mail, when Karin, a twenty-six-year-old Norwegian woman who had been blind since birth, came in and sat down at the opposite end of the room. I was so absorbed in my work that I didn't pause to greet her. After a few seconds she said, "Hi, Rose. How are you?"

I stopped typing and looked at her, extremely surprised. "Hi, Karin. How did you know it was me?"

"The sound of your typing." She was smiling her slightly crooked smile as she set up her computer. Her eyes were a bit sunken and completely unseeing. "Impossible," I said. "It could have been anyone at all sitting here typing."

"No," Karin said, grinning now, "it couldn't. You type faster than anyone on the campus. I always know when you're in this room from the sound of it."

Because it would never have occurred to me to analyze the sound of anyone's typing, because I never imagined I would be identifiable in this way, I felt weirdly naked and exposed. I asked Karin if everyone on the campus knew the sound of my typing. She shrugged. "Yes, of course."

One evening, one of the staff members gave me a coffee mug full of Indian beer, and though Paul and Sabriye discouraged alcohol on the campus, I thought it couldn't hurt for me to take the mug into the Internet room while I worked on my computer. I went into the crowded room, placed the mug carefully on the window ledge out of the way of any person who might come in and knock it over, and just as I was thinking, *Nobody will know there's beer here,* Gyentzen, at the farthest end of the room, said, "I smell beer. Who has beer for us?"

Again, I was astonished. "Gyentzen," I said, "you can smell a small mug of beer all the way down there?" Gyentzen laughed and confessed that he liked beer. (In his application to the institute, Gyentzen had described the Tibetan New Year celebration this way: "Homes are cleaned, new clothes are stitched, debts and quarrels are resolved, good food is cooked, and intoxicants are drunk.") Several other people in the room said that they too could smell the beer. I said, "Well, I'm sitting right on top of it and I can't smell it. What's the matter with me?"

"You are not a mystical blind person!" Jessica jeered.

As I made my way around the campus, I usually said hello to everyone I passed to alert them that I was there. But one night I was in a particular hurry to get back to my room and as I was going up the footpath, I saw Robbie, a German man who was completely blind, approaching me. Not wanting to stop and talk, I simply decided to pass by without speaking. What harm would it do if he didn't know who it was? But before I had got within thirty feet of him, Robbie said, "Hi, Rose."

I stopped in my tracks, baffled. "How on earth did you know it was me, Robbie?"

"The sound of your footsteps."

This one I found extremely difficult to believe. "Do you mean to tell me that of all the forty-some people who might be walking on this path tonight, you can actually differentiate the sound of my footsteps from everyone else's?"

"The shoes you wear have a particular sound."

I looked down at the shoes. They were simple sandals, just like the sandals of many of the other women on the campus. "Oh, for God's sake, they couldn't *possibly* have a particular sound," I said. I did not believe it.

"Yes, they do," Robbie said, "and you also walk faster than just about anybody here. I always know when it's you."

I was startled. If Robbie always recognized me, then probably everybody else did too. My fantasy of anonymity was destroyed. I understood once and for all that I could no more conceal my identity from a blind person than from a sighted person. I said good night to Robbie and continued on to my room, feeling transparent and vulnerable and wondering how many people I had insulted by passing by without saying hello. If they could identify me by the sound of my voice, I could understand that—I was capable of doing that too— but by the sound of my typing? The sound of my footsteps? The smell of my shampoo or soap or beer? What else was I unwittingly doing that my blind colleagues could identify as particularly *my* action and not someone else's? I was surprised that I hadn't anticipated how much the blind could know about me, what signals they received from my particular behavior, and by how intimate their knowledge of me sometimes seemed. Whatever Robbie knew of me, he probably knew effortlessly and without thinking about it. Because he was adapted to a sightless world, he was attuned to data and signals to which I myself was oblivious. Robbie and the others had noticed things about me that I had never stopped to notice about myself. This was not the result of some supernatural mystical ability or sixth sense, the kind of powers the blind have had pinned to them for ages; it was simply that the blind, like the rest of us, have a human need to recognize, to differentiate, and, above all, to connect with the people around them. My blind students knew me and connected with me in ways that I had never imagined possible.

When I asked my students to write an essay, I expected them to write it not in Braille but on a computer in an electric format that I could read. Braille is a beautifully useful tool for the blind, but since they were here to learn how to pass their ideas on to the world at large, which included a great number of people who were not blind, they had to know how to write effectively and type what they wrote on a keyboard. This was possible for blind people with a screen-reading program that read back to them what they had typed. The students who came from the more affluent countries—Japan, South Africa, and Europe—already had very good computer skills, could type quickly, and owned their own laptops. The rest either were still learning or had no skills at all. Occasionally I would go to the computer lab, an air-conditioned room in the classroom building with a bank of computers against one wall, and help the students as they wrote their essays. Those who already had good computer skills generally needed little help. They sat in front of the monitors, their fingers running quickly over the keyboards, while a flat electronic voice spoke their words back to them. (The voice was a speedy, monotonous babbling that sounded precisely like the muttering of a flock of farm ducks. It was a sound one heard all day long, all over the campus.) But the rest struggled, poking slowly at the keyboard with one finger, fighting with a cursor they didn't know how to control. Those who had a little vision tried, against the stern admonishments of Arky, the computer teacher, to actually read the letters on the keyboard and screen by pressing their faces to within an inch of them. Arky derisively called this "nose reading." Eric, a man from Ghana who had very weak vision on which he stubbornly continued to try to depend, would enlarge the font on his screen to an enormous size, then put his face to the screen and attempt to see it. Eric's eyelids had fleshy red growths at their edges and were generally swollen and sore-looking. He had no tear ducts, so he had to continually lubricate his eyes. It was painful to watch him struggling to see with these weak and damaged eyes. It was not only costing him a tremendous amount of time and effort but also preventing him from learning how to use the computer without sight, which eventually he would be forced to do, as his vision was ever diminishing. If he had simply closed his eyes and learned how to operate the computer without trying to see it, his work would have been much easier. But it is a monumental task to persuade a man to surrender a lifetime's pattern of behavior, a lifetime's identity as a sighted person, and get him to accept that he is blind. The English professor John Hull spent a tremendous amount of energy and psychic pain rejecting his blindness before he realized that "one must recreate one's life or be destroyed." The poet Stephen Kuusisto, author of *Planet of the Blind,* a memoir about losing his sight, described that process: "Why should it take so long for me to like the blind self? I resist it, admit it, then resist it again, as though blindness were a fetish, a perverse weakness, a thing I could overcome with the force of will power." By all accounts, abandoning life as a sighted person feels like a kind of death and yet the death is wholly necessary before a productive life as a blind person can begin.

The Liberian men, of course, had had no exposure to computers and were starting from scratch. The first essay that James typed on a computer looked like this:

0my personal experiesh on campux;on manuary w
　　2 19th 1
　　2009 , finding the treasure; on saturday janury 16th,participants
of the iise met in the auditorim

aut auditorim as usual. They were dicv
divided into four groups. A, v c
b,c and d to find a hidden treasure on the campux. Pr
ior to the treasure

And Johnson's looked like this:

Aaa social night a night that vrings eveeeery humanyring toghther
to asocial on january twelve came toghther for a dancebraillaaaaaae
with out yordersdid this beccause is custonary to dddo in culture
echangeto tekll you the ture this was .

Although there were enormous frustrations in the computer lab,
frayed tempers, and wounded pride, and although occasionally one
or another student would simply give up and walk out of the room
in a snit, they all persisted with the task. They sat at the computers
doggedly stabbing at the letters on the keyboards while the electronic
computer voices quacked it all back to them. In class, I often read
aloud the results of their writing efforts, and they were amused,
moved, and delighted by one another's stories, which inspired them to
write more. Sabriye proposed that we publish a school magazine (we
called it the *Spectacle*), and submissions for it poured in.

During their free time, the students occasionally walked to the bus
stop a quarter of a mile down the winding Nemom Po road and caught
the public bus into the city of Trivandrum. Of her first shopping trip
to the city, Pynhoi wrote in her all-encompassing, sweetly scattered
way:

Marketing When we talk about shoping i am so excited for it , then,i
count the things to buy ,i find that i have many things to buy . But
when i went to the market i enjoy marketing in different floor because

they sold different kinds of thing in every floor ,I also enjoy the stare which take me from the down floor to the top floor it is an electronic machine [escalator],I also enjoyed the bus cause they drived faster,the pinapple juice are really nice to have ,because the weather are hot but a bit expensive ,anyway i like it and i want to have it once more . As we came down to our campus by foot there are no electric as i came down i here different kind of birds and insects are making sounds .and i want some time to go inside the forest to just checked how they sleep but i am so afraied of snake so i desired not to go . When I reach back from the market and checked the things what what I brought from the market I find myself I only bought cream ,biscute ,pepsi .

Thank you from Pynhoi

In pouring out his troubles in his first essay, Gyentzen managed with his rudimentary English to express exactly what many of his colleagues had felt in their first few days at the institute. Martin's eyes filled with tears when he heard Gyentzen's comments about him:

tMy first time in the Camp My first day in the Camp is most unforgetable day for me in this year.

I heard many things about Camp in Kerala from Sbariye and Paul, but i never get feeling like living here. When i first come here i felt really quiet and nothing to do so depressed. In the night what i hear is sound of Birds and some other animal's sound and couldn't feel well…at that night i was afraid how to live here in Camp for one year. Because weather was too hot for me and together with i was home sick…and it was also a longest night for me…or i don't know how to say:

i had a terrible night at that day and i was thinking of my life in my country and couldn't sleep whole night. I wake up at the brake of down . But later it was getting better and i had a lots of fun with many different people. I knew there is water which we can swim and there are many place where we can do many defferent things and i went to swim one day witht some of our friends and i had a really nice day. Because sence i went to swim i felt not that hot when i first came here.

I got very nice guy with me in my room [Martin] and when i feel not happy he tells me lots of joke and always trying to makes me happy to be here. Also he told me we have to fight againest with our trouble....

And Khom got right down to the task of instructing sighted people in the ways of the blind with a wry, carefully thought-out essay entitled "How to Behave with the Blind":

By Khom Raj Sharma (Nepal)

If you are meeting a blind or visually impaired (BVI) person for the first time, you may wonder how to behave. The obvious advice is 'behave normally'. Here are some suggestions:

Please talk naturally. Don't talk down or address all your remarks to the person's companion as though the blind person were not there. Don't be afraid to say, "Nice to see you," for blind people say it too. When you approach a blind person and say hello, say who you are in case he or she doesn't recognize your voice. Address him or her by name, if you know it. If not, a light touch will indicate who exactly you are speaking to.

Before you move away, say that you are about to leave; anyone would feel foolish talking to an empty space. Persons with blindness and visual impairment may need your help. For example, many blind people appreciate being helped to cross a road or find a shop. If your offer of help is rejected, don't feel snubbed. The next blind person you come across will probably welcome your assistance. First, ask if you can help. Then walk slightly in front with the blind person holding your arm. If you are helping a blind person to get into a car, say which way it is facing and place the person's hand on the roof over the open door. If you are guiding a blind person on to a bus or microbus, you should go first. Never push the person in front of you.

Please inform the blind person if you are approaching a flight of steps or a slope, and always say whether it goes up or down. You should not worry too much about delicate furniture or ornaments, as most blind people move about without leaving a trail of destruction behind them. Show the blind person around the room and describe the furniture as you pass it, mentioning only hazards that are level with the head.

When a blind person is invited for a meal, he should be informed about the food being served. It is helpful if you describe for the blind the various sorts of food put on the plate in accordance with the location of the hours on a clock. For example: rice in the place of 12, Soup in the place of 3, vegetable in the place of 6, Meat in the place of 9 and so on. The cups or glasses should not be filled to the brim— very full cups are easy to spill. If you are serving a bony piece of fish, offer to de-bone it. Otherwise, your visitor will tell you if any help is needed; usually he or she will manage alone quite happily.

In class, we corrected the essays together and made suggestions for how to improve them. Class discussions had a way of turning to politics, social injustice, prejudice, ignorance, cultural taboos, ethical responsibility, and the challenges of social change. Students sometimes brought in selections from Braille books they liked and read them aloud. We read the *Times of India,* which was full of stories of bizarre domestic mishaps, murders, druggings, fatal bus accidents, and imperious letters to the editor about why women should not be allowed into Indian pubs and bars. (This last subject made the women in the class howl with outrage.) I read aloud from Ved Mehta's autobiography, *Vedi,* particularly about his experiences as a very young child at the Dadar boarding school for the blind in Bombay, and in the course of reading the story, I realized what an exceptionally good audience they were, how carefully they listened, how deeply they experienced what the words on the page conveyed. They murmured with disapproval and concern when something unpleasant or frightening happened to little Ved; they gasped and cried "Oh God!" in horror when I read that some of the blind children had died because of the poor health conditions at the school; and when they heard that Ved's mother blamed her son's blindness on the fact that his uncle had married an evil Christian, they laughed at the absurdity. They listened with complete absorption; the intensity of the expressions on their faces showed that in their minds they were actually living out Ved Mehta's experiences. Once or twice, Jessie was so racked with suspense that she spontaneously sprang up out of her chair. They enjoyed the story so much that word of it got around, and students who weren't even in my class began to come and listen. They loved picking up new words, like *shiftless* and *fickle, shabby* and *relish* and *shirk,* and phrases, like *perish the thought, to no avail,* and *kick the bucket,* and as soon as they learned these words and phrases, they began to use them in their daily speech with as much ease as if they had always known them.

Jayne and Lucy, two young Kenyan women who had gone to college together, were plump and talkative. They both had heavy Kenyan accents and an emphatic, declamatory way of speaking. They spoke Swahili when they were alone together, but their English was perfect. Jayne was a twenty-one-year-old red-haired, white-skinned African albino. When she was born, her face had been as white as the flesh of a banana, but over the years her forehead, cheeks, and lips had become mottled with large brown spots of melanin from overexposure to the dangerous Kenyan sun. Many albinos' retinas suffer from a lack of protective pigment, and Jayne's eyesight was extremely weak. She wore thick eyeglasses and spent a lot of time squinting and holding objects very close to her eyes. Although Lucy's skin was a rich dark brown, her mother was albino, and Lucy had inherited some of the traits of albinism—a large white birthmark under her arm and extremely poor vision. She, too, wore thick eyeglasses. She was twenty years old. Both girls were well educated and politically conscious, and both had come to the IISE because they wanted to start an organization in Nairobi to help improve the dire situation of African albinos and people with low vision.

One evening at dinner, they explained to me that in Africa, albinos were thought of as ghosts and were therefore believed to be in possession of magical powers. When a woman gave birth to an albino child, it was considered the result of a curse or some other form of bewitchment, and because of this, 70 percent of African albino children were abandoned by their parents. Jayne leaned close to me and said, "Some Africans don't dare to touch an albino, because they think that our white color is contagious. And lots of people believe that if you come in possession of an albino body part, you will have that albino's magical power in your control."

The high-ceilinged dining room at the IISE, which had a stage erected at one end and which doubled as an auditorium, was noisy at mealtimes. Groups of students and staff members sat at tables scattered throughout the large room, and the sound of multiple conversations, the scraping of chairs on the floor, and the clattering of cutlery crowded the room. I leaned closer to Jayne, the better to hear this strange story. Between forkfuls of rice that she squinted at minutely through her glasses, Jayne went on to tell me that an extremely lucrative black market trade in albino body parts had developed among the African witch doctors. "They kidnap and kill albinos like me so they can cut us up and sell our body parts. The fingers, hair, bones, skin, toes will be used to make magical charms and potions that promise to bring people power, love, long life, fame, and money. Last year in Tanzania, more than one hundred fifty albinos were killed and mutilated. We are hunted, I tell you."

Lucy, who had a slow, queenly bearing, a dry sense of humor, and a formal way of speaking, confirmed this fact by exclaiming, "Hey!" Then she put down her fork, drew a freshly pressed white hankie from the pocket of her flowered dress, and gently dabbed her perspiring brow with it. Even the Africans found Trivandrum unbearably hot. Lucy was pretty; she was also deeply conscious of her appearance and dressed with great care and style. That day she wore a blue flowered dress, a white Kenyan cloth wound proudly around her head like a chef's cylindrical hat, a blue necklace to match the dress, three white beaded bracelets, and a pair of black vinyl knee-high boots.

Jayne, too, was pretty and fashion conscious, but she was too impatient to spend excessive time on her appearance. She had a slow, forceful, confident way of talking, each word separated definitively from the next, and when she spoke, she never seemed to stop smiling, although sometimes I wondered if it was just her constant squinting that gave her round, speckled face the appearance of perpetual good humor. She had a habit of pedaling her hands up and down before her as she talked, raising her right index finger to hold her listener's attention, and enumerating facts by tapping the same index finger serially and dramatically against the tips of the fingers of her left hand. When she really wanted you to listen, she leaned close, put the palm of her hand flat against your shoulder, and held it firmly there until her point was made, whereupon she would stop talking, squint beadily at you, and let the hand sweep gently down the length of your arm. Finally, she would lean back and draw the pale hand toward her chest with a flourish intended to fix her words firmly in your mind.

Jayne told me that it was difficult for her to walk freely in the streets of Nairobi and that few people would want to hire her because she required protection in order not to be kidnapped and killed. She also could not take a job that required that she be outside in the direct sun. "So, my options are limited."

Jayne's mother had abandoned her at the hospital when she was an infant; it was her grandmother who took her home and raised her. "If not for my grandmother, I would be dead," she said. When she was in grade school, the other children wouldn't come near her. At thirteen she went to a national boarding school. "Nobody wanted to be with me there either," she said. "They called me hard words. I was outcast. I was either reading or in the chapel praying. Nobody wanted to sit with me." All the forty girls in the dorm had to shower together in one big open bathroom. Because Jayne didn't want them to stare at her white skin, she would wake up in the early hours of the morning, before dawn, shower alone, and then go back to bed. "One day I said to hell with it and I went to the shower with everyone else. As soon as I was naked, the whole school surrounded me and called me names. So I left the showers, put on my clothes, and did not go to class for two weeks."

There was one teacher at the school who defended Jayne, but that teacher soon left, and Jayne had to fend for herself. "Some girls would throw themselves in the nearby dam when they were frustrated or had troubles," Jayne said. "I was thinking to do the same. But I prayed. And I thought, *Why should I die because of other people laughing at me?*"

Jayne said that when she walked in the streets of Nairobi, she could hear people saying at the sight of her white skin and red hair, "That is good money passing us by now."

"Is it not despicable, Rose?" Lucy said.

The question needed no answer.

"They call us 'walking banknotes,'" Jayne said.

"And in Kenya," Lucy said, "they put people like us who have low vision in class with sighted students in school. It is an unfair practice."

"It was very hard for us to keep up in a regular sighted class. People with low vision need special facilities. But we had none!"

"None," Lucy said. Where Jayne was in the habit of raising her index finger to make a point, Lucy leveled hers sharply at her listener. "We fell through the proverbial cracks, as they say. The totally blind are better off in Kenya, because they get special attention. My mother faced a lot of discrimination because of her white skin and red hair. She worked in a school for visually impaired people. When I was young and could see well, I used to tease the blind children. I used to hide their white canes and dare them to chase me. Catch me if you can and the like! Little did I know then that I also had the gene for blindness. My sight deteriorated, and I had to wear spectacles. I wanted to become an airline pilot. Ha! Of course I could not. An engineer? Could also not. I must confess that when we went to college, we faced discrimination."

"Ahhh!" Jayne exclaimed in a confirming way; for Jayne and Lucy, *ahhh* and *hey* were completely interchangeable; they were both a form of *yes.* The two were as close as sisters and sometimes they spoke in contrapuntal harmony; at times, having a conversation with them was like having a conversation with one person graced with two mouths. They finished each other's sentences, spurred each other on, often disagreed for a few moments but then quickly swerved around to agreement again. They were fond of aphorisms and maxims, and occasionally they quoted from the Bible.

"The teachers told me I could not do science," Jayne said. "I was good at it, but they did not pay attention. They wrote on the blackboard, but I couldn't see what they wrote. I needed to hear what they had written, but they would not read it for me. I had to put my chair right up to the blackboard so that I could see the teacher's writing."

Jayne said she had studied very hard before her exams. She put her feet in buckets of cold water to keep herself awake at night as she studied. She opened the windows to let cold air circulate through her room. She knew math well but during the tests, she didn't have time to complete all the work. "They didn't give me large-type books or exams. It took me a long time to read the exam. In physics, biology, and chemistry I did well. The proof was in the pudding. But I got D minus in maths. I was good in maths, but I didn't complete my exam because I couldn't read it. They said, 'This girl did not go to special school, therefore we do not recognize her as visually impaired. Therefore, if she cannot do the exam, she fails.'"

Lucy defended Jayne by crossing her arms indignantly over her ample breasts. She shook her head vigorously. Her plump brown cheeks shone beneath the overhead lights. "Insensitive people, I tell you."

"And that teacher was a woman," Jayne said incredulously.

"A woman never knows to whom she will give birth."

"Ahhh. What kind of child will *she* have?"

"The quality of your life tomorrow depends on your thoughts today."

"I am sure that we will return to Kenya and change the life for the blind and the albino."

"Nothing ventured, nothing gained."

"We shall see what we shall see."

"God willing."

Jayne reached for her water glass, miscalculated its location, and reached a second time.

They told me about the street violence in Nairobi, the shootings and stabbings and robberies; the hijackers who posed as policemen at roadblocks and the thieves who climbed onto public buses, drugged all the passengers, and stole their wallets and jewelry. Once, while Jayne was in the dressing room of a Nairobi shop, a robber came in and shot the two Indian shopkeepers just as she was pulling a dress over her head. "I went out and I saw the two dead bodies and, oh, I was so scared, but I didn't look at them too long because I did not want to be a witness." I asked her why not. "Eh! I did not wish to become another victim!"

Lucy leaned close to me, her arms still crossed over her breasts, and in the firm, urgent tone of a mother dispensing imminently applicable advice to a child, she said, "Now, listen to me. In Nairobi, when you see a gun in the air, please fall down upon the ground immediately and ask no questions. Please do not look at them or sure they will shoot you. As for me, I prefer to fall on my stomach, because that way they cannot shoot me in the heart."

"Just let them shoot you in the rear end," Jayne told me with no trace of irony or humor.

"God forbid they should shoot you in the alimentary canal!"

"Or liver."

"Hey!"

In Kenya, the baddies would, apparently, kill you for anything—a cigarette, a spool of yarn, a bottle of beer. Jayne said, "In Kenya, you know, we leave our houses open. Not locked but open." She spread her legs to show me exactly how open. "The gangster, he will go right into any open house. This one gangster, he went into an open house and he told the man there, 'I have a gun! You take your pants off and you give them to me.' Then he set the house on fire."

Lucy clapped her hands over the table in disgust, then crossed her arms again and leaned back in her chair. "My boyfriend, he is a cop. He has a gun. Loaded at all times."

"To protect himself from you!" Jayne cried, and then she cackled for a good long while.

Lucy pursed her lips at Jayne. "Eh, wait until you have a boyfriend with a gun, Jayne!"

The Kenyan girls were street-smart, experienced, and not a bit shy about sexual matters, and yet they had quaint romantic fantasies and schoolgirl obsessions with the fairy-tale cliché of true and everlasting love. On the desk in her room, Lucy kept a Bible next to a smiling teddy bear with a floppy hat on its head and a bouquet of dried flowers hugged in its arms. They claimed to know all the necessary tricks of catching a man, pleasing him, keeping him awhile, and then dumping him on his ear when he turned out to be a no-good, selfish, two-timing, chauvinist chump, which without question he would turn out to be. They preferred blond-haired, blue-eyed white men to black men. Of Mohammed and Sahr, the two Sierra Leonean students, they said, "Eeee, those West African boys are too dark!" And when I said that I liked those dark faces, they told me, "White woman, you can have them!"

"The very dark men always seem to have glowing white teeth," I said.

Feigning boredom, Lucy sighed, examined her fingernails, fanned her ample cheeks with her folded hankie. "Okay, Rose, if there is a power cut, let them smile in the dark for you."

Jayne touched her lips in thought. "When they smile in the dark it is nice!"

Lucy squinted around the room, pushed her dinner plate away, and said to the ceiling, "In the dark they are all the same."

Not entirely off the subject, Jayne said, "Lucy has big breasts."

Lucy unfolded her arms to show me the breasts and said "Hey!" in proud agreement. "But you were never gifted in that way, Jayne."

"Ahhh," Jayne said ruefully.

"I wasn't either," I said.

Lucy looked me up and down through her thick lenses and then said pitilessly, "It is true. You are slight and without many gifts."

Since all decorum seemed to have gone by the boards, I mentioned the fact that Jayne and Lucy both had substantial rear ends. They liked this very much. Jayne said proudly, "Yah, Rose, if we carried a baby on our back, the baby would not fall off. Our ass would support him."

"Like a bookshelf, you see."

Jayne said suddenly, "The Pokot tribe in Kenya circumcise their cows."

"Cows?"

They collapsed in giggles. "They also circumcise their girls and put a bone in the entrance of the vagina to be removed by their husband on the wedding night. It is to keep the girl from going with other men. She does not have the desire."

"Is it not abominable?" Lucy said.

"Terrible," Jayne said.

Before we got up from the table that evening Lucy declared that the only good thing about blind men was that they could not see other beautiful women passing on the street in miniskirts.

Jayne raised her index finger. "Ahhh. But they cannot see you either, Lucy."

At some point during my stay at the IISE, a red-furred kitten showed up on campus and took up residence as the school pet. We called him Louis Braille. One day the kitten got into my classroom and ended up sitting on Victor's foot beneath the table. When Victor understood that it was the cat, he leaped out of his chair and shouted, "Oh, cat! Do not come around me!" He had moved so forcefully and suddenly that his big dark glasses fell from his nose to his lips.

I got up, put the cat out of the room, and asked Victor why he didn't want it near him.

Victor looked badly shaken. He straightened his sunglasses. "Auntie Rose, a cat can do witchcraft."

I dismissed this, but Johnson quickly defended Victor. "Respected Auntie Rose," Johnson said soberly, "in Liberia they use the cat for evil witchcraft. They would use this kitten. Because it is strongly believed in our setting that the cat is an ungrateful animal. No matter how much you care for it, it will betray you. Dog is submissive and obedient. Cat? Never!"

"I don't believe these superstitions," I said. "I don't believe in witchcraft." Approximately half the students said they didn't believe in it either.

Johnson, Victor, and James protested. "And dwarves also can do evil witchery," Victor said, "which is why they live only in the mountainous areas."

"Wait a minute, gentlemen," I said. "Tell me what a dwarf is."

Johnson said, "Dwarves are the small people in Liberia who live in the mountains."

I explained to those in the class who didn't know the term that dwarfism was a medical condition that retarded growth, that dwarves happened to be unusually small people with particular physical characteristics, and that there were dwarves all over the world, not just in Liberia. When I was sure that everyone knew what I meant, I asked the Liberians to explain what they were saying.

"Dwarves are frightening and dangerous and we stay away from them," James said.

"They are over in the forest," Victor said.

"They group together and talk among themselves," Johnson said. "They are human but they have a magical power. If you go near to them, you will never find a way out. They will grab you and tie you." Johnson made a keen grabbing motion with his small hands. "They live in the mountains, where all the diamonds and natural resources are to be found."

The men were not laughing. They spoke with conviction. They fully believed what they were saying. The very thought of these evil mountain-dwelling dwarves seemed to frighten them.

"They have natural magic, I tell you," Johnson said adamantly. "My people, God created them to make you disappear. They will make you dumbfound."

"Dumbstruck," Marco said.

"Dumbstruck, my brother Marco."

We sat in silence for a moment while the class tensely pondered the possibilities. Pynhoi teetered on the edge of her seat and peered nervously around the table, not sure what to believe. There were supernatural forces in her culture too. Kyila and Gyentzen, with their Tibetan fear of demons and spirits, also looked uncertain.

"So," I said. "You Liberians would not go near a dwarf, is that right?"

"That is right!"

"Have you ever met a dwarf?"

"We have not!"

"You have never met a dwarf and yet you believe all these superstitious stories about them. Is that correct?"

"Correct!"

"But isn't it true that in Liberia people also believe that blind people just like you can do evil witchcraft?"

"True!"

"Can you indeed do witchcraft?"

They were indignant. Victor raised his hands in the direction of my voice in a pleading way. "Auntie Rose, you know us. You know that we cannot!"

"But people who have never even met you believe that you can, in exactly the same way that you believe dwarves can without ever having met one."

A heavy silence followed. The ceiling fan buffeted the air above our heads. The day was overcast and oppressively hot; thunder purred faintly in the distance. The Liberians' faces were damp behind their

huge dark glasses. Jessie, who occasionally displayed mild characteristics of blindism, rocked slightly in her chair in a mood of coiled
suspense.

"Tell us why you believe these stories about dwarves," I said.

"People say them," James said.

"People say them because dwarves are physically different and that
scares them. Because they don't understand it. But people say the same
about you because you too have a physical difference. You're blind. You
know firsthand that what people say is not necessarily true. And those
false stories hurt you and make you angry. Isn't that right?"

All around the table, the students began to smile in recognition.
Jessie held up her hand and snapped her white fingers, an indication
that she urgently wanted to say something. She was smiling her foxy
smile and didn't wait for an invitation to speak. "Yah, so I think you
guys are doing to the dwarves the same thing what you don't want people to do to you. Ha!"

"That is called prejudice," Marco said, smiling.

"Discrimination," Kyila said.

I made the point that prejudice and discrimination most often
spring from irrational thinking and unfounded hearsay. The Liberians
sheepishly pursed their lips. Finally Johnson conceded that we might
be right.

I said that if the Liberians brought a mountain-dwelling Liberian
dwarf into the classroom and staged a witchcraft competition between that dwarf and one of our magical blind colleagues, and that
if I could witness the outcome of that unusual competition, then I
*might* believe their stories. "Otherwise, much as I love you, I think
you are three collaborators in a social tyranny. The worst part is, you
don't even know it."

They knew that I was teasing them and laying it on thick. They also
knew that what some of us were saying made sense. They had con-

structed a wall between dwarves and themselves for reasons that did not hold up under scrutiny. I suggested that this was where justice and reason ended and evil began and that facts, evidence, and truth were the only antidotes to the damage that superstition could do. Whether their ingrown, inherited animus toward dwarves would ever change was anybody's guess.

As I was leaving the classroom that day, Victor came to me and said, "Auntie Rose, one question: Are you African American?"

The question took me by surprise. "No. I am white. Why are you asking me that?"

Victor said, "We thought you were African American."

"But why?"

"Because one day you read us a poem by an African American woman."

The poem was Maya Angelou's "Human Family." At Sabriye's request, the other teachers and I had read it to our classes. The last line of the poem is "We are more alike, my friends, / than we are unalike."

"That's a funny reason to think I was African American, Victor. If I had sung you a Chinese song, would that make you think I was Chinese?"

Victor smirked and said nothing, and we all made our way down the hall. Perhaps he had had enough logic for one day. I began to sing "Dong Fang Hong" ("The East Is Red"), a famous Communist Chinese song, and Gyentzen, who was walking behind us and was well versed in Chinese propaganda from a lifetime spent in Tibet, recognized the song and began to sing it with me.

Some days when it was particularly hot, we held our classes on wooden benches beneath the shade of the coconut trees at the edge of the lake. The breeze that picked up there in the afternoons offered the only relief from the unbearable heat. One afternoon, the seven members of the school literary magazine and I gathered at the lake to review recent student submissions. Jessie and I were the official editors of the magazine, but that simply meant we did the typing, the organizing, and the nagging when a submission was past deadline. The editorial board also included Yoshimi, James, Victor, Karin, Eric, and Holi. Since I was the only sighted person, it was often left to me to read the submissions out loud from a laptop screen. I enjoyed doing it, and I particularly enjoyed it when the others laughed at something in an essay that amused them. Once, I had to read aloud a very short piece that Johnson had written about his early life, and at the beginning of the last paragraph, a sudden flood of tears prevented me from reading further.

> ...My Child Youth Days
>
> From the time my mom gave birth with me, along with my twin sister, she found it very difficult to meet our daily meal, because she was left alone with the children without a husband...She was two months pregnant when daddy left for the United States of America, and never returned up to now...mom decided to send us to a primary school near the town when I was twelve years old. it was one afternoon, at 2:15 PM, my twin sister called Zennah experienced a hot fever for one hour and could not feel any part of her body if she is touched. In this light, I suddenly lost my only twin sister on may 3, 1985, while at the age of thirteen. When I was promoted to fifth grade in 1988, again this time around my mom got seriously ill on June 6, which lasted for two months and she again died on August 8, 1988.
>
> Why this happened to me again? What I have done to you, God?

There was more to this essay, but I was so impeded by unexpected emotion that I had to stop and return to it later. Johnson's loss of his mother and sister, his plea to God, struck me as doubly moving because not once in his essay did he mention the fact that he had lost his eyesight to an exploding bomb at the age of twenty-one and that as a result his remaining family members had abandoned him; it was as though that major detail in his life was inconsequential compared to the deeper injury of losing his mother and sister. Too, his preoccupation with the specific dates of these sad events was characteristically Liberian and seemed to me to underscore his suffering.

Submissions to the magazine included fiction, personal essays, world news, current events, articles about our responsibility toward the environment, information on open-source software for the blind, ethnic recipes, and jokes. That afternoon we critiqued each piece and discussed how to improve it and whether it was worthy of publication. As we talked, the breeze transformed the surface of the lake from a flat plane to a chaos of serrated ripples; the edges of the lily pads flipped upward at its force. The lily pads were big enough that full-size coots could walk across the water on top of them. I could see, far off across the lake, two men poling themselves along in a wooden canoe. Terns cruised low over the water. Down to the west, a baby water buffalo stood among the reeds at the edge of the lake with a black crow pecking at insects on its back. A bird in the trees behind us screamed. A neckless, chestnut-brown kingfisher with an electric-blue back and a beak like a letter opener sat hunched on a palm frond above us, casting a murderous eye over the water. I could see smoke rising above the palm trees at the agricultural college on the other side of the lake. As Jessie began to offer her opinion on a particular piece, I noticed, from the corner of my eye, a tiny twitching in the long grass just to the right. Something was moving low along the ground in the grass between us and the lake. I turned my head and realized that it was a large snake weaving toward us at a slow, steady pace. I was transfixed, afraid to move. When the snake got to within twenty feet of us, I stood up. It was a grayish-green color with a yellow underside and a bluntly rounded nose, like the toe of a businessman's wing-tip shoe.

"Everybody, please get up and move away toward the auditorium," I said. "There's a big snake coming toward us."

They closed their laptops, got up unhurriedly, rattled their canes into the straight position, and stayed where they stood. At the sudden noise and motion, the snake, too, stood up. It lifted the front part of its long body several feet off the ground, straight as a staff, and looked at us. And then, before my eyes, it flexed its head into that unmistakable spoon shape that I had seen a thousand times in films, but only in films. It was a cobra. In films, that hooded head always looked terrible and real and close. This cobra was real and close, but because I had never seen one before, it looked somehow inauthentic. In reality, it looked hokey and unreal. It was almost literally unbelievable, like an illusion that would evaporate if I rubbed my eyes. I watched it in frozen fascination and disbelief. I saw it but did not quite accept it. It was like a bad joke. All it had to do now was open its hard, lipless little mouth and show me its forked tongue and venomous fangs, and the joke would be complete. I had a strong and inappropriate impulse to laugh, to say, *Oh, come off it!* But this was not a zoo or a film. I had to accept the fact that this was Kerala, a hot, jungly place "recognized as having a major problem with snakebite," a place where one had to battle the wildlife in one's own bedroom. There was no expert here to protect us or charm the snake down with a bamboo flute. The cobra's bite has enough venom to kill twenty human beings. Since I was the only one here who could see it, it seemed to fall to me to protect myself and my blind students. I came to my senses. The voice of my human education said, *Run.*

"It isn't just a snake," I said. "It's a cobra. Please, all of you, *move.*"

At this, a few of them lifted the tips of their canes off the ground, but still they did not turn and leave. Why weren't they running away screaming, the way I was on the verge of doing if they didn't hurry up and *move?* They just stood looking puzzled and apprehensive and even a little bored. I began to push and herd them off, saying, "Go! Now! Move back to the buildings immediately!"

When they heard the distress in my voice and felt my hands on their backs, they began to skitter and stumble up the footpath. The noise frightened the snake, of course, and it disappeared into the grass. I stood on the path staring at that spot in the grass, waiting for it to return or for some other unbelievable creature to emerge. I was afraid to look away, but I had to in order to see where my class had ended up. They were huddled at the top of the footpath, silently clutching their canes and facing in five different directions. I knew that if they had been able to see that snake, they would not have been standing there like that. They would have been long gone and safely indoors. But most of them had no idea what a snake looked like, let alone a cobra. All they knew was that snakes were something that sighted people found deeply disturbing. They had to take our word for it. But then I too had had to take someone's word for it. Never having been bitten by a snake or strangled by a boa constrictor, I had had to take someone's word for what those creatures could do to me. Many of the things that sighted people fear, we fear not from firsthand experience but because we've been warned. It is no different with the blind.

I looked back at the grass, regretting that I was the only one who had seen the famous, awful, unbelievable creature. And what sighted person would believe that I saw it? Who would believe a fabular story about a bunch of blind people being chased by a cobra? It made me feel lonely to realize that I had no fellow witness. As frightened as I was, I was delighted to have seen it and a little disappointed that the snake was gone. I looked from the grass to the students and back. Was it safe to sit down there again? I wasn't eager to risk it. "Well, okay. I think he's gone," I said. "Let's just go to a classroom and finish our work."

As we went up the path, the Africans eagerly offered advice about how to keep snakes away. "Put garlic around the lake!"

"Spray Cuprinol on the grass!"

"Burn a lorry tire nearby! They do not like that rubber smoke, it is said."

"Yes," I said, "but neither would we. Just beat the grass with your white canes the next time you come down here, and the snakes will run off. They're more afraid of you and your canes than you are of them."

One Saturday afternoon, a couple of other teachers and I organized a class trip into the city on the public bus. The bus stop was a quarter of a mile away from the campus, on the main road. Eight or nine students and two teachers, Nora and Isabel, and I set off down the narrow Nemom Po lane on foot. Nora was German, and Isabel was Spanish and French—both were smart, extremely hardworking, empathetic, and strong. Robbie, who had traveled a great deal in his life and who was comfortable navigating in unknown surroundings, led the pack with his white cane. Robbie had lost his vision to a brain tumor when he was not yet two years old, and his father had abandoned the family. He was highly intelligent, a bit of a loner, a talented and imaginative writer, and, after living in Ireland for five or six years, where he worked for a radio station, he spoke English every bit as well as I did. Like Jessie, the other German student, Robbie could be moody: one minute laughing and eagerly participating, the next minute defensive, superior, sullen, and aloof. He had long frizzy hair that he parted in the middle. His face was soft and pale and fleshy, and in repose he sometimes looked woeful and beset. His eyes appeared completely healthy, but his eyelids often drooped in a way that made him look drugged. He had a reddish mustache, a small shapely mouth, and very red lips. Robbie was tall and nearly as thin as Gyentzen, with long legs, a high waist, and a short torso. He often adopted the Indian style of dress, wrapping a paisley-patterned cotton cloth around his waist instead of wearing trousers, and on his feet he wore black rubber Crocs. The Indian skirts exposed his pale thin legs. Of all the students at the institute, Robbie had the most impressive scars on his shins, perhaps a result of his fearless eagerness to venture into the world, move about, and have adventures.

James and Johnson followed behind Robbie that day, their white canes examining the pavement. It pleased and amused me to see these two big family men holding hands as they walked, with their heads lifted high, as if to smell their surroundings. Behind them, Yoshimi and Victor, also with canes, walked arm in arm. Yoshimi was pretty, olive-skinned, petite, and had long thick glossy black hair cut in blunt bangs across her forehead, a style that seemed to me quintessentially Japanese. She was fond of frilly blouses, short skirts, and modest high heels. Yoshimi's eyes were pinched shut most of the time. She had plump round cheeks and smiled easily, revealing strong, evenly shaped white teeth. She was brilliant, capable, diligent, always good-natured, versed in all the latest computer technology, and after studying for one year in the United States she spoke English better and with less of an accent than any Japanese person I had ever met. Arm in arm, little Yoshimi and the enormous, nearly unintelligible Victor were a highly unlikely pair. I wondered as I walked behind them whether they would have been walking so easily together if they had been able to see each other. They were good friends.

Khom, who had forgotten his white cane, walked behind Gyentzen with his hand on Gyentzen's shoulder. And Lucy and Jayne straggled at the rear in broad-brimmed hats. They walked in an ambling way, talking all the while.

As we passed through the village, local people working in their yards dropped what they were doing, came to the edge of the road, and stared. When was the last time they saw a parade of blind people walking down their little road? And not just blind but African,

Japanese, albino, Tibetan, Nepalese, and European. The sight was so unusual that some of the local children backed away as we neared, and one very small one burst into tears. A man and wife came out of their house to watch. The man pointed at his own eyes and said to me, "Blind school?" I said, "Yes." A barefoot woman smiling tooth-lessly and carrying a bucket of earth on her head sat down on the raised root of an enormous banyan tree to watch us go by. A couple of chickens skittered across the road in front of us. Crows glided in and out of the mango trees. The road was overhung with tree branches, palm fronds, impossibly tangled electrical wires, and vines of bougainvillea. Farther along, a little girl standing at the gate of a house watched us for a while, went into the house, and came back out with another girl, and they both stood at the gate, staring with their mouths open. An old woman who had been crouched on the ground hacking at a palm frond with a crescent reaper dropped the reaper as we approached and stood up to stare at us with her hands on her hips. She smiled; her teeth were stained dark orange from the betel nut she was chewing.

The students walked on undisturbed. They could hear the locals speaking the Malayalam language to the left and right along the way, and certainly knew they were being watched, but this was nothing new to them.

At the bus stop, we sat on the bench and waited in the sickening heat. Yoshimi had brought a paper fan and fluttered it before her face. Jayne fanned herself with her hat and said, "It is better on campus be-cause of the breeze from the lake. The breeze cools down things when things are heated up."

Lucy stared straight ahead and said in her poker-faced way, "When are things in Trivandrum *not* heated up, Jayne? Eh? They are heated up all the time, Jayne. How are things now? Cool? Are they cool?"

Jayne fanned Lucy with the hat. "They are heated."

Lucy dabbed her forehead with her ever pristine hankie and said, "Hey! Is it not true?"

Side by side, Jayne's and Lucy's arms contrasted as sharply as black and white chess pieces. I could feel the heat wafting up from the pavement beneath our feet; it was like the heat from a pizza oven with its door flung wide. I had to stand up and pace back and forth to get away from it. Barefoot Indians walked languidly up and down the roasting road. Motorized rickshaws, taxis, motorcycles, bicycles flew by in a noisy tangle, thoroughly ignoring the fact that in India, vehicles are supposed to drive on the left. A bus whose sign read *Ananthapuram Fast* bounced by, followed by a yellow school bus with *Little Flower Convent School* written on its side. After that came the Mar Georgis EM Church bus, the English medium school bus, and a dump truck with *Christ Jesus* painted on its front in bright colors. Once a fertile breeding ground for missionaries, the city of Trivandrum was full of Christian churches of every imaginable denomination, some of which I had never heard of, including the Syro-Malabar Christians of Saint Thomas.

We climbed onto the Trivandrum city bus and sat amid the sleepy passengers nodding in the heat, and the bus careered its way into the city.

Once we arrived, we walked from the bus stop to Big Bazaar, the main department store in Trivandrum, and the students dispersed through the aisles, eagerly touching everything on the shelves. The store was new and, relative to every other store in Trivandrum, quite modern; it had one of the few escalators in the city. Most of the students rode happily up to the second floor on it, and Lucy and Jayne in their enormous hats rode up and then down again for fun, but Victor refused to go near it. "Is that an electric stair?" he asked me, clutching his white cane with one hand and feeling the moving handrail with the other. I said it was. "Oh, I do not want that one," he said. "That thing will make me feel unoriented and throw me down." I tried to coax him onto it, told him I would hold his arm and be sure he didn't fall, but it was no use. He was dead set against anything that might take his feet out from under him. I asked him which he was more afraid of, a cat with supernatural powers or an escalator.

"Auntie Rose, do not joke!"

Victor was so adamant that I relented and led him up the conventional staircase at the back of the store.

That day Victor wore a sleeveless orange basketball shirt with the number 17 on its back and front; walking among all the small Indians, he looked, except for the white cane, like a professional basketball player on holiday. People jumped out of his way when they saw him coming. Victor went gleefully through the store selecting more merchandise than he could afford. And he was fussy about his purchases. He wanted skin cream and soap. "But," he said to me, "I want them to smell nice." He stood in front of the shelf of bath soaps and sniffed at eight different brands, rejecting them one by one until, finally, he selected the most expensive. Then he picked up a blue polo shirt, spread it against his chest, and said, "What color is it?" I told him. "Does it suit me?"

"Beautifully."

"Are you sure, Auntie Rose? Because I like to look nice."

"You look great."

That satisfied him.

Lucy and Jayne passed by us, squinting and smiling. Jayne put her face to mine, raised her index finger, and said, "Rose, this store is not good. They have more men's clothes than women's."

"Yah," Lucy said, and added in her deadpan way, "they are gender-insensitive."

Jayne slapped her thigh. "And the Indian size underwear is too small for us!" They hee-hee'd a lot at this and then drifted on.

After forty-five minutes of exploration, of laughter, of knocking merchandise off the shelves, of trying on Indian clothing and sniffing

Indian produce, the students gathered at the registers and made their purchases. The Indian staff were surprised and fascinated by them but polite and very helpful. When we went out onto Mahatma Gandhi Road, I was amazed to see James plunging alone across the wildly busy avenue with his white cane raised over his head to command the traffic to stop. I watched him with my heart in my throat. The traffic was extremely dense, but the drivers had no choice but to bring their vehicles screeching to a standstill while James passed through with his head held high, like Rosa Parks sitting at the front of the bus. He reached the far sidewalk and stood there for a minute or so, listening to the traffic, then he raised his cane again in an authoritative, declarative way and stepped back into the street. The traffic stopped once more, and he crossed safely back to us. As he approached the sidewalk, I took his arm and said, "James, what on earth are you doing?"

"In Liberia," he said, "that is how we cross the street. I just wanted to see if it works in India."

"It would probably work anywhere. But it's not the best way for anybody, blind or otherwise, to cross an Indian boulevard. Next time you want to cross the street, promise me you'll just go to a corner and cross on the crosswalk like everybody else!"

When I turned around, I saw Robbie standing statue-still in the middle of the sidewalk holding a digital device at arm's length in order to record the cacophony of noises in this soot-colored city. A crowd of young Indian men with tight jeans and slicked-back hair had gathered near him to stare; they looked completely puzzled by the sight. With his skirt and his wild hair and his pale white face and long scarred shins, Robbie the German was in some ways a more striking sight than the Liberians. The young men were snickering at him; Robbie either didn't know or knew and didn't care. As far as he and James were concerned, Mahatma Gandhi Road was theirs.

# Sight Regained

Reading the case study of a twelve-year-old congenitally blind Parisian girl who, in 1850, suddenly came to understand the nature of sight, I was struck by how accurately the girl's perceptions and feelings defined the aspect of blindness that I would fear more than any other. After having the power of sight described to her, the girl devised an experiment whereby she might test what she had now come to suspect about sighted people. She got up one morning and put on an old dress that had become much too short for her growing body and that, consequently, she had not worn for some time. Without saying a word, she entered a room where her sighted governess was working. Upon seeing the girl, the governess expressed surprise that she had put on the old dress that "only reaches to your knees." The girl uttered a few "idle words" to the governess and left the room. Later she stated:

> This was enough to convince me that, without laying a hand upon me, Martha had immediately been able to recognize that I had again put on the dress that was too short. So this was seeing. I gradually recounted in my memory a multitude of things which must have been daily seen in the same fashion by the people about me and which could not have been known to them in any other way. I did not

in the least understand how this happened, but I was at last persuaded. And this led gradually to a complete transformation of my ideas. I admitted to myself that there was in fact a highly important difference of organization between myself and other people; whereas I could make contact with them by touch and hearing, they were bound to me through an unknown sense, which entirely surrounded me even from a distance, followed me about, penetrated through me and somehow held me in its power from morning to night. What a strange power this was, to which I was subjected against my will, without, for my part, being able to exercise it over anyone at all. It made me shy and uneasy to begin with. I felt envious about it. It seemed to raise an impenetrable screen between society and myself. I felt unwillingly compelled to regard myself as an exceptional being, that had, as it were, to hide itself in order to live.*

These feelings, among a host of others, would be my sentiments exactly if I were blind and had never known sight. *They can all see me from across a football field and thus know a thousand things about me, but I can't see them and cannot know a damn thing about them without going right up and putting my hands on them.* It would frighten and irk me exactly as much as if I were unable to walk down a street briskly and with ease. The vulnerability and the imbalance of power would infuriate me; it would gnaw at me; it would make me come to dislike myself a great deal and make me dislike sighted people a great deal more. I too would want to hide.

Although the girl's reaction seems to me entirely justified, her negative response to her understanding of sight is not one that the blind often express; in fact, in my extensive reading about blindness and

---

*Von Senden, *Space and Sight*, 61.

the experiences of the blind, I came across only one other similar statement. (In his memoir of his blindness, John Hull spoke of wanting to hide his face from other people. "Is this a primitive desire to find some kind of equality? Since your face is not available to me, why should my face be available to you?" But he also addressed the unique way in which the blind could make the sighted feel inadequate: "The disabled person tends to render other people powerless. One flusters them, covers them with confusion, covers them with uncertainty and embarrassment, makes them feel gauche and insensitive, awkward and intrusive.") And, surprisingly, not once have I ever heard an acquaintance who was blind—congenitally or otherwise—speak with resentment or unhappiness about this particular imbalance in the powers of perception between the sighted and the blind. No blind person I have ever met has expressed to me any displeasure at all over the fact that sighted people can see the blind while the blind cannot see the sighted. (Many, however, will freely express resentment at the prejudices the sighted visit upon them.*) This doesn't mean they don't think about the sighted having this power or feel a discomfort about it similar to the French girl's; it just means they don't tend to bring it up. Or perhaps they don't bring it up with sighted people. Further, the

---

*In his memoir *Planet of the Blind,* the poet Stephen Kuusisto did say that as a blind person, "you are watched everywhere you go," and that as a watched blind person, he sometimes felt "buried beneath the graffiti of other people's superstitions." Yet, after years of sufferring caused by his trying to pass as a sighted person, Kuusito finally chose to present himself to the world as a proud, self-directed blind man, and in doing so he found that "there's power that comes with admitting how little I can see because the world is more open and admits me far more graciously that it did when I was in the closet." The blind author Georgina Kleege pointed out that there was discomfort on both sides. While the sighted were indeed in a position to observe the blind freely, they also tended to feel a vulnerability and powerlessness in the face of that persistent myth about the supernatural powers of the blind. "They seem to secretly suspect an unseen force prompting our responses...extra accurate hearing and perfect pitch...a finer touch, a bloodhound's sense of smell. We allegedly possess an unfair advantage that we could use against the sighted, hearing the secrets in their sighs, smelling their fear."

majority of those congenitally blind whom I directly questioned about whether they would want to gain their sight if it were possible said that they were happy as they were and would prefer not to acquire that fifth sense. I can attribute this only to the fact that most of them have lived successful, contented lives without sight for so long that its sudden advent would be superfluous, and perhaps even disruptive. Sabriye, who was in some ways happier with her life as a completely blind person (as opposed to a partially sighted person), had turned down a chance at corrective surgery for the same reasons. When I asked Yoshimi Horiuchi, the twenty-six-year-old Japanese student, if she would want to regain her eyesight (she lost it at approximately age five), she said vehemently, "Never!" When I asked her why, she said, partly in jest, "I would never want to be a part of the whole corrupt sighted racket!"*

For people who were born blind or who lost their sight at a young age, the prospect of gaining sight rarely inspires the excitement and joy that those of us who already have it would naturally expect. The congenitally blind who have fared well and been comfortable all their lives with what their four senses have been telling them can certainly be forgiven for not jumping at the chance to change it all by throwing the mystery of eyesight into the equation. They have no way of knowing whether eyesight would be, for them, a curse or a gift. The unknown and the inexplicable are not immediately appealing.

The fact is that suddenly gaining sight is not the miraculous revelation we might suppose it to be. In almost all of the known case studies, those people who have surgically gained sight after a

---

*Yoshimi had a good sense of humor and liked to joke, but she explained for me a general political resentment that many blind people have: the fact that the world is organized, philosophized about, and run according to the needs, terms, and demands of the sighted, while the needs and views of the blind are largely ignored. It is a resentment of the sighted people's presumption that their perception of reality is the only perception. For Yoshimi, that was a corrupt racket.

lifetime of blindness have inevitably found the experience psychologically disturbing, confusing, and dispiriting. In a representative case in Vienna in 1777, a fourteen-year-old congenitally blind girl who had regained her sight through surgery expressed her eventual despair in words strikingly similar to those uttered by many others who found themselves in precisely the same position: "How comes it that I now find myself less happy than before? Everything that I see causes me a disagreeable emotion. Oh, I was much more at ease in my blindness... if I were always to feel such uneasiness as I do at present at the sight of new things, I would sooner return on the spot to my former blindness."

The human infant is not born with useful vision. He is born with eyes that see but a brain that does not yet know how to process the visual information the eyes transmit to it. What the infant sees makes no immediate sense to him; the world appears a brilliant chaos of light, shape, and motion. Learning to see is one of the most difficult mental tasks we accomplish in a lifetime; in that process, the brain is taxed perhaps more than it will ever be again.* Vision is a slowly acquired skill that depends wholly on physical experiences combined with the type of exceptionally malleable and receptive neurons found only in a very young brain. The brain learns to make sense of what the eyes are showing it in a complex process similar to the way one learns to speak, and it learns all of this during a period of great flexibility—the first seven to ten years of childhood. Once that period of receptivity has passed, it cannot be retrieved or re-created. A newly sighted person can adapt to his rudimentary vision and use it to his advantage, but he

---

*"Each eye sends the brain a billion messages per second. Together the two eyes transmit twice as much information to the brain as the rest of the body combined" (Georgina Kleege, *Sight Unseen*).

cannot learn how to see with the thoughtless, carefree facility of those who have always had sight.

In 1020, a man named Ammar recorded the case of a thirty-year-old congenitally blind man whose sight was surgically restored. Since then, there have been remarkably few cases of sight restored to a person who had been blind since birth or who lost sight at age three or younger, a condition known as lifetime blindness. In his unique and unexpectedly moving book *Space and Sight: The Perception of Space and Shape in the Congenitally Blind Before and After Operation,* which was first published in Germany in 1932, the German scientist Marius von Senden collected all the available case studies of patients whose sight had been surgically restored. On the evidence of these cases, von Senden concluded that a person born blind who gained vision at a later age could not develop a truly useful conception of shape, form, or depth. Most could perceive color and motion with relative ease, but all other visual tasks proved extremely confounding.

As an example of the formerly blind person's inability to comprehend space and size, von Senden told of a sixteen-year-old French girl who, when asked to show her doctor how big her mother was, "did not stretch out her hands, but set her two index-fingers a few inches apart." Similarly, a twenty-year-old Swiss man who had gained sight for the first time could not "imagine a great distance in any other way save in terms of the time one has to spend walking in order to get there.... He sees contours and colors; but when I talk to him about a very long distance, it does not seem as though he can imagine any such thing." In 1728, the thirteen-year-old whose cataracts William Cheselden had removed understood that "the room he was in ... [was] but part of the house, yet he could not conceive that the whole house could look bigger." In another case, an American woman named Joan could conceive of a skyscraper only as being "indefinitely higher than a blind man can reach." On first gaining vision, one man had to practice spatial distance and depth by taking off his boot, throwing it ahead of him, and then trying to gauge how far away it was. "He takes a few steps towards the boot and tries to grasp it; on failing to reach it, he moves on a step or two and gropes for the boot until he finally gets hold of it." Von Senden remarked that even after some weeks, the same man still had no concept of space beyond what he saw directly before him. "He does not yet have the notion that a larger object (a chair) can mask a smaller one (a dog), or that the latter can still be present even though it is not directly seen."

In all the recorded cases of vision restored, the subjects have had excruciating difficulty making sense of human faces. This passage from the case of a thirty-year-old Scottish man who has just opened his eyes after surgery is virtually identical to the experience of many others: the patient can guess that he is looking at a face only because he hears a voice coming out of it:

> The first thing he actually perceived was the face of the house-surgeon. He says that at first he did not know what it was he saw, but that when Dr. Stewart [who was bending over him] asked him to look down, the sense of hearing guided his eye straight to the point whence the sound came, and then, recalling what he knew from having felt his own face, he realized that this must be a mouth, and that he must be looking at a face.

One surgeon tested his sixteen-year-old patient's vision by inviting her beloved uncle to come silently into the room and sit by her bed. The surgeon then positioned himself behind the uncle and asked the girl to look at the face before her. She did so and immediately informed the surgeon that the face she was looking at was his own. When he invited her to put out her hand and feel the face, "she stretched out her forefinger and ran it over a quite small surface of her uncle's cheek, and immediately her face beamed and she cried: 'It's my uncle!'" The surgeon who operated on Joan, the American woman, stated that, postsurgery, "faces are so bewildering to [her] that she still judges people by their voices."

Almost all of these patients were incapable of identifying three-dimensional objects by sight alone and were compelled to stretch out their hands to feel them, whereupon they would recognize the objects instantly. They would, for example, know a fork by feeling it, but if they saw it lying on a table, they would have no idea what it was until they touched it. Cheselden's patient had a pet cat and dog; on gaining his vision, the boy could see them but could not tell which was which. He would pick up the cat, know it by touch, and swear that the next time he saw it he would know it was the cat. But no matter how many times he practiced with the two animals, he repeatedly mistook one for the other. According to Cheselden, the boy "learned and forgot a thousand things in a day." Similarly, the twenty-year-old Swiss patient was unable to identify objects on his first day after surgery, leading his surgeon to assume that the operation had been a failure. On the second day, the patient was shown a watch and was able to identify its color but could not say whether it was a square or round object until he was allowed to hold it in his hand, and he then immediately knew that it was round. Again and again all the physicians' experiments revealed the same thing: the newly sighted patient could determine color and motion but could not make sense of any form until he was allowed to touch it.

Distance and depth perception prove to be equally confounding. When the anthropologist Colin Turnbull spent time with Pygmies in the Amazon rain forest, he came to understand that their experience of living in the dense jungle limited their visual perception of distance. Since the vegetation in their environment was never more than, say, ten feet away, their visual understanding was necessarily limited to a distance of ten feet. When Turnbull drove out of the jungle and into wide-open space in the company of a Pygmy man who had never before left the closeness of the jungle, he was astonished to realize that his companion had no understanding of the vast distances he was looking at. At the sight of buffalo grazing a mile or two away in an open valley, the Pygmy asked Turnbull, "What insects are those?" In *The Forest People,* Turnbull wrote:

> At first I hardly understood; then I realized that in the forest the range of distance is so limited that there is no great need to make automatic allowance for distance when judging size.... When I told Kenge that the insects were buffalo, he roared with laughter and told me not to tell such stupid lies.... As we got closer, the "insects" must have seemed to get bigger and bigger.... [Kenge's] only comment was that they were not real buffalo, and that he was not going to get out of the car again until we left the park.

One newly sighted patient believed that a table at the center of a room was really flat against a far wall, and several others defined a sphere as nothing more than a circle, and a cube as nothing more than a square. In a case in Italy in 1846, a patient was asked to take an orange that was held in front of him, and he gravely miscalculated its position, raising "his hand so that it almost touched his eye, and then clenched his fist, which he was astonished to find empty." Joan had a poetically surreal perception of the world around her: a black coat on the floor looked to her "like the mouth of a well," smoke from a chimney looked like "a great crack in the bright sky," and the spots on her dog, Muffy, looked like "alarming holes in him." Paintings and pictures also made little sense to the newly sighted, appearing as patches of color; the patients who touched the surfaces of pictures were astonished to find that the images were flat. When presented with a realistic painting of a table laden with food, one patient jumped up and nearly poked his hand through the painting, and when it was explained to him that the images he saw were painted on a canvas, he "had to be suffered to convince himself of the fact by repeatedly feeling with the greatest care the length and breadth of the painting." When Joan was given photographs and paintings, she asked, "Why do they put those dark marks all over them?" Her mother explained to her that the dark marks were actually shadows. "If it were not for shadows, many things would look flat." Joan responded, "Well, that's how things do look. Everything looks flat with dark patches."

All the studies have shown that the experience of newfound sight is extremely difficult. A young man who regained his sight in London in 1840 found walking the city streets "disagreeable and wearisome" and "tedious" because too much of what he saw he couldn't understand.

> He said, seeing so many different things and the quick movements of the multitude of people, carriages, etc., confused his sight to such a degree that at last he could see nothing; that the sensation produced by the object last seen had not yet disappeared from the retina, when the next object made its impression thereupon, by which means confusion of ideas, great anxiety, even vertigo were occasioned, from which he could only free himself by closing his eyes for a few moments.

This young man's experience was similar to many other patients'. One boy, accompanied by his sister, was upset by a ride on a tramcar. At the sight of houses passing rapidly before his eyes outside the tram window, he remarked, "I don't like that at all. It's going too fast." And at the sight of the many wares in a shopwindow, the boy expressed nothing but bewilderment. A French surgeon wrote of his sixteen-year-old patient, "She obviously found the untried experience of seeing somewhat disturbing; and how gladly did she receive permission to close her eyes."

When they tried to see the world, the patients generally saw a riot of shapes, colors, and motion untempered by sense or reason. Some found their first impressions beautiful and fascinating, but the euphoria was often quickly replaced by fatigue and apprehensiveness. Most suffered serious psychological crises, lost their confidence, and fell into depression, despair, and disillusionment. Many longed to be once again blind. In 1826, a forty-six-year-old London woman confessed on the sixth day after her surgery that her vision had improved since the previous days, "but I cannot tell what I do see. I am quite stupid." Her surgeon averred that "she seemed indeed bewildered from not being able to combine the knowledge acquired by the senses of touch and sight, and felt disappointed in not having the power of distinguishing at once by her eye, objects which she could so readily distinguish from one another by feeling them." The patients didn't realize that their own brains were preventing them from making sense of what they saw, and it's no surprise that these patients became disappointed, frustrated, and depressed. Surgeons didn't understand that asking their patients to see fluently postoperatively was essentially no different from asking them to speak a foreign language fluently—Icelandic, say—when they had never studied it before. The Austrian surgeon Georg Joseph Beer, who restored sight to fourteen people between 1783 and 1813, stated that all of his patients suffered a "rapid and complete loss of that striking and wonderful serenity which is characteristic only of those who have never yet seen.... Gloomy and reserved, they now shun for a time the society of others, which was so indispensable to them while they were blind." Indeed, many who became despondent simply closed their eyes and reverted to their blind way of life.

*    *    *

One of the most in-depth case histories of sight regained was con-
ducted by the British psychologist Richard Gregory. Gregory's study,
published in 1963 in the *Quarterly Journal of Psychology,* was the first
of its kind since 1904.* The subject, Sidney Bradford, was a fifty-two-
year-old cobbler who had become blind at the age of ten months. By
Bradford's own account and by the accounts of his sister and teachers, although he could see some light, he had never had useful vision
and spent a great deal of his childhood with his eyes bandaged.† Before his surgery, Bradford had lived a well-adjusted, relatively active,
and quite fearless life as a blind man. He rode a bicycle with his hand
on the shoulder of a companion riding next to him; he engaged in car-
pentry with power tools in his shop; he painted his own house, a task
that required him to climb ladders. In 1958 Bradford underwent a
corneal graft operation and regained his sight. On meeting him forty-
eight days after the operation, Richard Gregory observed that at first
he appeared to be like any other sighted person, but when Bradford
sat down in a room, Gregory noticed that he did not look around the
space with any apparent curiosity or recognition and that he paid no
attention to material objects unless "his attention were called to them,
when he would peer at whatever it was with extreme concentration
and care, finally making some almost oracular comment."

Gregory was surprised when Bradford looked at a large clock on

---

*The details and outcome of this case are remarkably similar to those of the case of a man
named Virgil, whom Oliver Sacks studied in 1991 and wrote about in his book *An Anthropologist on Mars.*

†Again a distinction should be made between the profound blindness of those who have
completely unresponsive retinas and the blindness of those who cannot see in any useful
sense yet do have vital retinas that can perceive some light. Sight can be recovered only if
the retina is vital.

the hospital-room wall and read the time, and he began to think that perhaps Bradford had not truly been blind before. But Bradford explained his ability by showing Gregory a large watch without a crystal covering it that he had previously read by feeling its hands. He said that since he had felt the position of the hands, he could now understand what they indicated just by looking at them. With color he was less adept and was able to identify only red, white, and black—colors that he claimed had been stored in his visual memory. He was also unfamiliar with the appearance of faces, unable to recognize them and unable to read facial expressions. Bradford told Gregory that when he first opened his eyes after the surgery, he heard a voice near him and turned his head toward it. Like the Scottish patient, he understood that the blur he was looking at must be a face, because a voice was coming out of it; without the voice, though, he would not have been able to identify what he saw as a face. Gregory wrote, "At the time we first saw him, he did not find faces 'easy' objects. He did not look at a speaker's face, and made nothing of facial expressions. On the other hand, he very rapidly distinguished between passing lorries and cars and would get up at six each morning to look at them some way off." Gregory surmised that Bradford's interest in vehicles derived from the fact that they made familiar sounds that helped in their identification.

Bradford had difficulty judging distances, and when looking down from a window forty feet high, he believed that he could lower himself from the window to the ground. Later, standing outside on the ground and looking up at the same window, he understood what a great distance it was and how dangerous it would be to step out of it. Three days after his surgery, Bradford saw the moon for the first time and thought it was a reflection on the windowpane. When told it was the moon, he was surprised and fascinated to see that it had a crescent shape; he had expected a quarter moon to be shaped like a quarter of a cake.

Gregory noticed that Bradford, like many people in his position, was reluctant to admit mistakes in his perceptions and was uncomfortable expressing surprise at certain phenomena in his newly sighted life. When presented with various geometrical optical illusions printed on paper, Bradford failed to see the illusions, which Oliver Sacks in a similar case attributed to the fact that his brain had only a "rudimentary" ability of visual construction, a direct result of his not having had enough visual experience at the beginning of his life. Looking at pictures, Bradford had great difficulty identifying what they contained and had no idea whether a particular object lay in front of or behind other objects. In his own drawings of objects, Bradford could not include any object that he had not previously touched with his hands; his conception of the world had been formed by touch, a conception that was nearly impossible to alter.

Once Bradford was released from the hospital, his mood predictably declined. Driving in a car, he was unresponsive to the scenery that passed by, because, he explained, it moved too quickly for him to understand it; he also seemed to find the appearance of the world "drab." When Gregory took him on a tour around London, Bradford appeared bored; he was uninterested in the buildings and was drawn only by moving objects. As a blind man, he had crossed busy streets by himself with complete confidence and without the aid of a cane, but now that he could see, he refused to try to cross by himself, and even when led by a sighted person, he expressed uncharacteristic fear. Gregory wrote, "We began to see that his assurance had at least temporarily left him; he seemed to lack confidence and interest in his surroundings."

Because Bradford had an interest in tools, Gregory thought that a visit to London's science museum would lift his spirits. Looking at the famous Maudslay screw-cutting lathe within its glass display case, Bradford had no idea what it was and could correctly identify nothing but the handle. His inability to recognize the parts of the machine frustrated and upset him. It was not until the lid of the glass case was opened and Bradford was allowed to run his hands over the machine that he could make any sense of it. Once he had felt the device to his satisfaction (with his eyes closed) and understood it, he declared that having felt it, he could stand away from it and his eyes would now be able to see it. In order for him to really see, information had to be transmitted through his hands first.

Gregory took Bradford to the zoo at Regent's Park, where Bradford was able to identify roughly half the animals by sight; the other half he couldn't name, in some cases because he was unfamiliar with the animal. Bradford was highly amused by the sight of two giraffes looking down at him from over the top of a fence, and on this Gregory remarked, "This was the only visual situation noted which ever made him laugh." Bradford responded well to the animals, seemed to enjoy touching them, and he was able to toss cabbages to the hippopotamuses with accurate aim. (And yet when Gregory engaged him in a game of darts—which Bradford had played when he was blind—it was determined that his newfound vision had no significant beneficial effect on his dart game.) Gregory's general observations after spending two days with Bradford were that he could walk down a staircase with confidence and ease without holding the banister but that if the flight of steps was short, he was inclined to step off the top step without anticipating the rest. He could also walk directly past an object eminently worthy of notice—an elephant, for example—without seeing it at all, and yet when asked if he could see Big Ben from outside Buckingham Palace (a distance of perhaps a quarter mile), he was able to see the tower. "He only looked at faces when spoken to," Gregory wrote, "and then in a rather 'blind' fashion, though there was some evidence on the second day that he was beginning to look at faces with more curiosity. At a meal, one would look up and find him rather tentatively studying one's face."

Six months after the surgery, Gregory made another visit to Bradford in his home and found that he seemed "dispirited" and that his sight seemed to be "almost entirely disappointing." Eyesight had not given him the opportunities he had imagined it would. He continued to perceive the world around him as drab and stated, "I always felt in my own way that women were lovely, now I can see them I think they're ugly." Bradford told Gregory that more and more he had begun to notice the "blemishes in things," and he would fixate on these blemishes or irregularities with consternation and distaste. The physical world did not live up to his imaginings of it. He was puzzled also as to why things seemed to change shape and appearance as he walked around them and viewed them from different angles.

Gregory concluded that Bradford's exhaustion and his disillusionment with his newly restored vision had led him to return to his life as a blind man. At night, he often did not turn on the lights in his house, because he was more comfortable in the dark. He had poor relationships with his neighbors, who "regarded him as 'odd,'" and at work he was teased for being unable to read despite the fact that he now had sight. Gregory determined that Bradford's vision recovery had been psychologically damaging and had cost him his self-respect. Previously, he had appeared to his acquaintances a happy, powerful person. Now, Gregory wrote, "it seemed to all of us that he was deeply disturbed; yet too proud to admit or discuss it." After some time, Bradford's wife wrote to Gregory to tell him that Bradford had been ill with "internal shingles and nerve pain" and that he was "disappointed about everything." Five months later she wrote to say that he had not improved. "I wish you could help him. His nerves are so bad. I can see his hands trembling even as he ate his porridge this morning, and he could not cut even sausages on his plate.... I want to get him well again, as he was a cheerful help to me and lots of people, and he had great faith and patience, which has now gone. It seems to me our world is not as grand as we thought, and Mr. B did not know the way people acted—until he got his sight."

Nearly two months later, at the age of fifty-four, Bradford died. Richard Gregory wrote of him:

> His story is in some ways tragic. He suffered one of the greatest handicaps, and yet he lived with energy and enthusiasm. When his handicap was apparently swept away, as by a miracle, he lost his peace and his self-respect. We may feel disappointment at a private dream come true: SB found disappointment with what he took to be reality.

The most recent case of sight regained in a person with lifetime blindness is that of Mike May, who, after being blinded at age three by an accidental explosion, acquired sight in 2000 in an experimental corneal epithelial stem-cell transplant. With his book *Crashing Through: A True Story of Risk, Adventure, and the Man Who Dared to See,* Robert Kurson gives a detailed report of May's case. By all accounts May was, though blind, a fearless child. He ran about and played games like any other child; he roller-skated, skateboarded, rode a bicycle with the assistance of friends. In high school he rode a motorcycle around a track, and, later, he took up downhill skiing, which he managed to do with the vocal guidance of a coach who skied alongside him. May skied so well he won international downhill competitions for disabled skiers, skiing with the tips of his skis eighteen inches behind the skis of a sighted guide in front of him, who led the way with commands. Eventually May married, had two sons, and founded an innovative technology company.

After much careful deliberation, May decided to go through with the pair of surgeries that his doctors believed would restore vision to his eye. (He had only one eye; the other one had been removed years earlier due to an infection.) The surgeries were a success, and when the bandages were removed from his eye, he could see. Like Bradford and so many other patients, May was able to see color and motion very well but was unable to recognize faces or make sense of facial expressions. In fact, people's facial movements and expressions were so distracting to him that he had difficulty concentrating on what they were saying and felt he had to close his eyes in order to really listen to them. Kurson writes of May: "When the women spoke their heads bobbed, their lips flapped, their hands gestured. This bedlam at once amused and distracted him, and try as he might he could not keep track of what they were saying, so long as their faces ran spastic like that." Faces held no meaning for May, and all faces looked the same. He could not tell his sons apart by looking at their faces. He could distinguish the letters of the alphabet but had a hard time reading. A flight of stairs looked like nothing more than a set of horizontal lines, and on a walk to a local doughnut shop with his guide dog, he had trouble differentiating the rise of a curb from the street and nearly tripped over it. The only step he was able to see and anticipate was a step down near the doughnut shop, which he had learned to expect. He found it difficult to differentiate shadows from solid objects. He could see clearly a line of cereal boxes on a supermarket shelf but couldn't separate one box from the next. He began to feel frustrated that he could determine color easily and catch a ball easily and yet couldn't tell who was male and who was female when he sat in a coffee shop and looked at the customers' faces. Like Bradford and countless others, May could be certain he was identifying an object correctly only if he felt it with his hands.

After he had had vision for six weeks, his wife asked him how he felt about it. May answered, "It seems like I have to process every little thing consciously to understand what I'm seeing. Everything is interesting to me, but sometimes it feels like I can't do anything in peace."

He had to think very hard to make sense of what he saw. Every new object, he had to study and work at to understand. And like Bradford, May was disturbed when he saw aspects of the world that appeared ugly to him. Garbage in the street, cracked windows, and a homeless person lying on the sidewalk upset him inordinately. Like most newly sighted people, May found his vision was better when he was in familiar environments. When he saw the television remote control lying in its usual place on the coffee table in his house, he recognized it, and yet if the remote appeared in an unexpected place, he could not say what it was. After four months, he began to find his restored vision overwhelming and exhausting. He worried that this would continue for the rest of his life.

The only difference between Bradford's story and May's is that the fields of ophthalmology and neuroscience have advanced enormously since 1959, and in the year 2000, May's case presented an invaluable opportunity for ophthalmologists and neurologists, who were aided by the latest medical and technological innovations. Kurson writes, "Today it is virtually impossible to find a vision scientist, researcher, or psychologist who does not agree that knowledge and vision are highly related, and that without our knowledge about the visual world, our ability to understand visual scenes would fall apart." He goes on to explain that an infant learns how to see the world by interacting with it, by touching whatever appears before him, by grabbing it, putting it in his mouth if he can, exploring it with his fingers, drawing it closer and pushing it farther away. Touch and vision inform each other, and without this partnership of constant practice and experiment, it is impossible for the human brain to learn to make sense of what it sees. In the same way, the ability to distinguish one human face from another and to comprehend subtle facial expressions comes only after much repeated exposure to faces, which infants and young children experience every day. To human beings, one monkey's face tends to look pretty much like any other monkey's face, although, as Kurson points out, one monkey's face differs from the next to essentially the same degree that one human's face differs from the next. The reason we can't make the distinction is that most of us have no experience interacting with monkeys. "Children are still developing their face-perception skills at five or six years of age," Kurson notes. Humans have much early practice, so the gift of seeing becomes automatic; as adults, we don't need to think about or work at it. If the neurons meant for vision aren't used at an early stage of development, they learn other tasks, but they lose their flexibility and cannot later revert to their original purpose. Magnetic resonance imaging of May's brain during an array of visual tests confirmed that the areas of his brain that should have been recognizing faces and objects simply did not respond to them. Kurson succinctly frames the basic problem behind May's—and, indeed, all the newly sighted patients'—confused vision: "It was likely he would never perceive faces, depth, or objects normally because he, like all adults, no longer had the available neural networks to learn them."

In 1606, when the philosopher William Molyneux asked his friend John Locke if he thought that a person born blind who had learned to distinguish a cube from a sphere simply by touching them with his hands could, upon regaining his sight, distinguish the two simply by looking at them, he was essentially asking whether sight regained (or, more accurately, *first* gained) in a blind adult would be an instantly effective tool. Locke surmised that it would not be. The question was debated for centuries. With Mike May's case, the question has been definitively answered. Those who do not have the early childhood experience of seeing and interacting will not, if they gain sight in adulthood, know how to see.

# The Definition of *Real*

L ate one afternoon I was sitting at the desk in my bedroom at the institute when I heard some of the women returning from a shopping trip into the city. As they mounted the stairs to the second floor of the dormitory, their heads were momentarily level with the front window of my room, and Lucy took the opportunity to shout, as she always did, "Rose! Your girls are home!"

Yoshimi was asleep in her bed with a bad cold; I stepped out onto the walkway to tell them not to wake her, but it was too late, they had already burst into her room to see how she was. I went in to find Jayne giving Yoshimi a rough pat on the forehead; Yoshimi sat up, and in the process, her thermometer fell from the bed to the desk. Jayne groped around the desk until she located the thermometer, held it up to her eyeglasses to see what it was, and suddenly the thermometer emitted a few words of Japanese in a loud electronic voice. Jayne was so startled, she jumped, but when she began to comprehend what it was, her surprise turned to delight. "Eh!" she cried. "Yoshi's thermometer speaks Japanese!"

Lucy grabbed the instrument from her and examined it in the window light. "And it has Braille on it," she said.

"Ho! I never saw that before," Jayne said. She gave Yoshimi a little shove on the shoulder. "Oh-la-la. Techno Japan is ahead!"

Yoshimi smiled and blew her red nose on a hankie.

Jayne turned and put her face close to mine. "Japan is ahead of everybody, eh, Rose?" She had just eaten a cookie or a biscuit; I could smell the sweetness of it on her breath. Around her neck she wore her dorm-room key on a string. She was wearing sandals, and I saw that she had painted her toenails. The terrible thought came to me that in Nairobi, each one of those pretty white toes had a monetary value.

Standing at the foot of the bed were Holi; Karin; Yoshimi's roommate, Kyila; and Chelsea, a blind Indian girl who had been working in the office of the institute. While Kyila's side of the room was always tidy and orderly, Yoshi's side was a riveting mess. Her desk was piled high with handbags, clothes, candy wrappers, computer equipment, Braille books, and electrical wires. Her closet doors were flung wide, and clothes spilled out onto the floor. There were stray shoes scattered everywhere. Her white cane lay crumpled by the leg of her desk. Once, when I commented on the disorder of her room and the fact that blind people usually like their surroundings to be neat, Yoshi replied that for her the room was perfectly organized, that she knew the location of every single item and rarely had to search for anything. One day I saw her pulling clothes from her drawers and dropping them onto the floor, and when I asked her why, she said, "So that I can separate the dark from the light so I can wash them." I didn't ask her how she could tell the dark from the light. I knew her well enough to know that she had probably memorized the feel of every item, and once she had been told its color, she retained it in her memory. Another time, I had run into her in the laundry room, where she was ironing some of her clothes, and when I praised the detailed embroidery on one of her handkerchiefs, she asked me what the word *embroidery* meant. I explained it to her and ran the tips of her fingers over the stitching. "Oh, that," she had said. "Yes. Is it nice?"

"It's a very pretty outline of a horseshoe."

Yoshimi seemed surprised. "It is?"

"You didn't know that?"

"No," she said. "I could feel it, but I didn't know what it was. My older sister, she is six years older than me. She chooses most of my clothes and things for me, but she doesn't say much about them."

I remarked that her sister must have very good taste, because Yoshimi was always nicely dressed.

"My sister never tells me I look nice in my appearance. Well, once I cut my hair a little bit different and she did say it was nice. But that was all."

That seemed strange to me, and mingy. I said, "Well, probably your sister is just envious of you."

Yoshi laughed loudly at that. As I was leaving the laundry room, she lowered her voice and said, "Rose? I found a pair of...well, a pair of...things that we wear under the skirt in my laundry, and I know that they do not belong to me. I don't know what to do with them." She seemed extremely embarrassed to be bringing this up.

"Those things are called underwear."

"I know that," she said, ducking her head, "but I don't like to say that word."

"It's just a word, Yoshi. We all wear it. It's not shameful." Yoshi was a bit innocent and very sweet; she had told me that she cried every time she saw *The Sound of Music* and that she knew all the words to every song in the film; she'd also said that one of her favorite songs in English was "If You're Happy and You Know It, Clap Your Hands," but still, I hadn't realized she was so prudish. Certain that I was about to send her into a tailspin, I said, "Well, the best way for you to return them to the person who owns them is to make an announcement about it in a general assembly."

Yoshimi nearly had a heart attack. She clapped her hands over her mouth, then threw them full force in my direction, then hopped up and down in front of the ironing board with her hands squeezed into fists and her black bangs trembling, then screamed in protest: "Ohh! My God! Rose! Are you *kidding* me? I could never do that!"

I told her that if she was too shy to do it, I would be happy to make the announcement for her.

"Okay," she said. "Announce it. But, God, *please* do not mention my name or anything about me to do with the...the things!"

Now Yoshimi was lying sick in her bed with the bawdy, freewheeling Jayne and Lucy ministering to her. Yoshimi had taken to calling Jayne and Lucy the Kenyan sisters, and because Yoshi was so technologically advanced, the Kenyans referred to her as Techno Jap. Beside her pillow, Yoshi had set up a little shrine of Japanese Buddha figurines. Jayne had found them and was now making them dance the Watusi on the mattress.

Chelsea came around from the foot of the bed with her white cane, tripping on shoes and clothes as she did, and declared happily to me that they had all just come from the city, that she had guided them in and back without mishap, and that she had even haggled with the bus driver over the price of their tickets and they had got away with paying only eight rupees per person.

"But," Lucy said with admiration and envy, "Chelsea paid nothing."

"Because," Jayne said, "she is Indian and has a government pass."

I said that I wouldn't mind having a government pass, and Lucy agreed, backhanding my arm and saying, "Hey!"

Chelsea, who was a rather literal person, stated that I was not eligible for such a pass as I was not Indian and not blind.

Chelsea was twenty-four and had been completely blind since birth. She was born in Chennai to an upper-class family and spoke elegant English with a slight stutter and an extremely refined accent. She was small and slender and, in my opinion, the best-dressed person on the campus. Every morning she appeared at breakfast in yet another freshly washed and pressed traditional Indian outfit in a colorful pattern, with a flowing silk scarf around her neck and her short black hair styled sleekly against her head. She wore gold bangles on her wrists, small gold earrings, and pretty necklaces. She exhibited several distinct blindisms, including an occasional flicking of her fingers as she talked, a slight wagging of the head, and a habit of pressing her thumbs against her eyelids when she was concentrating carefully on something. Now and then, I saw her talking to herself under her breath, but I certainly could not attribute this to blindness, as I often did the same.

Chelsea's mother had died when Chelsea was very young, and now she lived in Trivandrum with a hired woman whom she referred to as her maid. Her upper-class upbringing had given her a strict set of codes, manners, and rules for life. She would never wear trousers in public unless she was accompanied by someone she knew well. Her grandmother, who was English but lived in America, had sent her a Jackie Collins novel; Chelsea had deemed certain explicit scenes "too hard to handle." Her father was a Sikh who not only cut his hair short but did not wear a turban; she disapproved of this unorthodox behavior. In addition, the father, who spent a lot of time in Thailand, had girlfriends. Her relationship with him was rocky because he had, as she put it, a double standard. When Chelsea told me that she had a boyfriend, I was surprised, as that didn't seem to fit the upper-class pattern. Young men and women were not allowed to mix until they were married. Chelsea later emended the term *boyfriend* by noting, "Well, I should say he is not actually a boyfriend but a boy who is a friend, and actually I have not seen him in three years. We talk on the telephone. My father hates this so much. He does not want me to have a boyfriend, even though he himself has girlfriends. Sometimes he recorded my telephone calls with the boy and said he would have the boy's mum dismissed from her job if we talked again. So, it is a double standard."

I told Chelsea that it was not just a double standard but a gross interference in the lives of three people.

Chelsea said that her father's extreme overprotectiveness was due in part to her blindness, that most things in her life had been done for her, and that even now her maid and her father continued to tell her "You can't do this; you can't do that." When she met Sabriye, Chelsea was amazed at how much Sabriye was able to do for herself. "I never saw a blind person being so assertive and independent in my life."

Chelsea had already learned a great deal from Sabriye and the other blind students. Leading the shopping expedition into the city was clearly a point of great pride and satisfaction for her. She was delighted that others had trusted and relied on her. And she was finding her own voice. When we made a visit to the government grade school for the blind in Trivandrum, Chelsea came along. The mustachioed principal of the school, a well-intentioned but passive and inarticulate man with a potbelly and strands of hair combed over his bald spot, had been completely blinded as a child after he fell out of a coconut tree and hit his head. In a grim classroom with a concrete floor, plywood doors, one fluorescent lightbulb hanging crooked on the wall, and great cobwebs clinging to the beamed ceiling, the principal told us that the school had only twelve Braille typewriters for fifty-four students and that the government was very slow in providing them with the proper Braille books for their curriculum. But all in all, he said fatuously, his blind students did not face any problems in the world beyond his campus. "Most people in society are eager to help the blind." The clock on the wall behind him said 6:45. It was in fact 10:55. When asked about mobility training and the use of the white cane, the principal said, "In Kerala, blind people think that a white cane marks them as inferior. I myself have stopped using it because I was becoming dependent on it."

I could see my blind students shaking their heads in disapproval at this, and quite unexpectedly Chelsea stood up and roundly chastised the principal in both English and Malayalam, saying that blindness was not a curse, that blind people were not the same as sighted people in certain respects, and that to downplay that was to ignore an important difference. "You want to be seen as a normal person in society, so you won't allow yourself to benefit from the use of the white cane. But blind people should be *proud* of their white canes. We should be proud of our blindness and not try to hide it." Chelsea, of all people, had boldly articulated what everyone else was thinking.

The sound of sweeping and the burbling Malayalam conversation of the cleaning ladies drifted up from the courtyard below Yoshimi's dorm room; a bird let out a sharp wolf whistle, and then fierce barking came from the back of the building. Chelsea cocked her head at the sound. "When a dog barks, it signifies death."

Karin the Norwegian said, "We say that if a dog howls it means earthquake." The barking continued. "Rose," Karin said, "I have been meaning to ask you, what exactly is the view from our dorm windows at the back of the building?"

I was surprised by the question. I knew the students so well now that I tended to forget that they couldn't see. I went to the back window of the room and began describing the view to them. Beyond the wall of the institute, which was close behind the dorm, was a large lot of coconut and mango trees. At that moment at the end of the lot, two small cows stood tethered to a tree, and, closer to us, two men were raking mango leaves into a pile with tiny brooms made from twigs. Just to the right of them, three boys were hacking at the trunk of a mango tree with machetes. One of the boys I recognized, as he was often in this lot with his mother. In fact, the mother was now approaching the boys with a twig broom in her hands. She wore a long loose gown and what looked to me like an entire bedsheet wrapped artistically around her head. The boy, who was not more than eight years old, could climb a coconut tree with the ease of a monkey. He was so skinny that he looked almost weightless. His legs were like a spider's. Many times I had seen him shimmy barefoot up the shaft of a coconut tree to a height of at least fifty feet with his machete tucked into his belt while his mother stood impatiently watching from below, her hands on her hips and the broom tucked under her arm. The boy would draw out his machete, brace the soles of his bare feet against the trunk and hug it with one arm, and hack at the fronds of the palm until they plummeted to the ground, whereupon the mother would gather them up and drag them away to a hut at the far end of the lot.

"What do they want the palms for?" Karin asked.

"I have no idea," I said. "But it must be important, because the boy often risks his life to get them. Also, sometimes when he's at the top of a tree, he tries to look through our windows."

All the girls gasped in alarm. I reassured them that he probably couldn't see much.

Holi said, "I smell smoke."

She was right—the two men had set the pile of mango leaves on fire, and the smoke was just beginning to curl over the institute wall.

Yoshi said from the bed, "Something is always burning out there."

"Oh, and I hear the announcement," Karin said.

We were all familiar with the announcement. It was a loudspeaker connected to a truck that roved through the villages of the area exhorting the people to fight polio by availing themselves of free polio vaccines. Every few weeks, the polio truck would creep along the Nemom Po road through the palm trees, loudspeakers blaring with alternating male and female voices. On this day, the polio truck was followed by what I had come to think of as the ice cream bike: a man dressed like Gandhi riding through the village on a bicycle with a basket of cones attached to its front and a box of ice cream attached to its rear. Children trailed after him.

I went on describing what I could see from the window—the ice cream bike, the children, the men with their brooms—and finally Yoshi said, "It must be very beautiful."

I turned from the window, slightly taken aback and at a loss as to how to respond to this. While the view here had certain small charms, I would not have classified the place as beautiful. But the perception of beauty is subjective. Did my vision give me greater authority in assessing whether the place was beautiful? Sight was one thing—sensibility was another. In saying the place must be beautiful, Yoshi seemed to be deferring to my sighted opinion, bestowing on me an authority that I didn't feel I had a right to accept. I didn't think this place was particularly beautiful, but many people did.* And I was curious to know how she and the others perceived their surroundings before I contributed my interfering and not entirely appreciative perspective. They must by now have created an image of their environment. "What do you think?" I said. "In your mind, is it beautiful?"

Propped up in her bed, Yoshi said yes, she thought it was beautiful. She based this on the sounds she could hear (the birds, the babbling of the turkeys and the lowing of the cows, the Indian voices, the rattling of the palm fronds in the wind) and on the things she could feel (the coconut trunk and its long fronds, the smooth mango leaf, the cool lake water, the feel of the movement of the air). She had determined that the place was beautiful; the others had too. Their sightless perception was as real to them as my sighted perception was to me.

In her book *My Path Leads to Tibet*, Sabriye had written about this question.

What's the definition of real? Does it mean that, for sighted people, reality is limited to what their eyes see? Is priority accorded to visual

---

*As Hamlet tells Rosencrantz and Guildenstern, "There is nothing either good or bad, but thinking makes it so."

impressions, which overwhelm the other sensory perceptions?...If the eyesight is "privileged"—as is the presumed case for those who can see—are we implying that the other senses do not contribute to the total perception of reality?

I once asked Jessie, blind since birth, how she imagined human faces. Her quick response was "I don't." A person's face was not, for her, the locus of an individual's being. Physical appearances were irrelevant. She turned her attention to the voice, to the words it created, to the mood and the ideas it formed, and this was fully satisfying for her. She and her blind colleagues lived in a realm dominated by thought rather than appearances and visual details. John Hull, the British professor of religion who lost his sight in his forties, went through a period of great despair and difficulty over the loss. But eventually, after a tremendous emotional struggle, the despair passed, and he entered a phase of his life that to me, pointlessly preoccupied and distracted as I am by every little visual detail before me, seemed pure and clean and almost enviable:

> There has been a strange change in the state or the kind of activity in my brain. It seems to have turned in upon itself to find inner resources. Being denied the stimulus of much of the outside world, it has had to sort out its own functions and priorities. I now feel clearer, more excited and more adventurous intellectually than ever before in my life. I find myself connecting more, remembering more, making more links in my mind between the various things I have read and had to learn over the years. Sometimes I come home in the evening and feel that my mind is almost bursting with new ideas and new horizons.

Hull summarized this experience by saying that as a blind person, "one begins to take up residence in another world."

\*     \*     \*

A month and a half into my stay at the IISE, Aias, my boyfriend, came to visit me for a few hours. Not having spent time with any blind people before, Aias was not entirely comfortable with my blind colleagues. I could see his discomfort in the way he shook their hands, in the way he talked to them—or seemed not to know how to talk to them—and in the way he had to work to hide his unease when he looked at their eyes. Their blindness struck him uncharacteristically silent. And when we had left the school and gotten on a bus to the city, he said to me with concern and disturbance in his voice, "Those poor people. What a life!"

"Do you feel sorry for them?" I asked.

"Yes, of course I do," he said.

"But they don't feel sorry for themselves. They're strong and happy and very capable. You just don't know that yet. You don't *know* them. Because they've accepted their blindness, it can't stand in their way. They've found a way around it."

"But they can't see anything," he said in frustration. "They're missing so much. And they're helpless and vulnerable to everything."

Aias offered that he would rather die than be blind. I understood his perception, of course. I had felt the same thing. For most of us, vision is the primary way we interpret the world, the most elementary, and so how could we connect and identify with a person who cannot see? We take our physical health and integrity so much for granted and rely so heavily on it that those who don't have it seem alien and pitiable. I remember being surprised by a statement that the British writer Geoff Dyer made in *The Missing of the Somme,* his compelling book about the Great War. In describing the mute impassivity and vulnerability of the many British war memorials, figures of soldiers in bronze and stone that stand forever subject to the whims of vandals, graffiti artists, and the elements, Dyer wrote, "Powerless to protect themselves, their only defense, like that of the blind, is our respect." I remember thinking how perfectly the comparison encapsulated the age-old cliché that having no eyesight is tantamount to having no brain and therefore no power. Dyer, an extremely intelligent, perceptive, and talented writer, had, like so many people, overlooked what the blind have most in common with the sighted: they are capable of thought. And unlike figures of bronze and stone, they can speak for themselves. In matters of the blind's self-defense, sighted people's respect for them is irrelevant. The blind can well enough defend themselves. Aristotle posited in *Rhetoric*, "It is absurd to hold that a man ought to be ashamed of being unable to defend himself with his limbs but not of being unable to defend himself with speech and reason, when the use of rational speech is more distinctive of a human being than the use of his limbs." Since it is the human brain and the human heart that differentiate our species from animals, since it's the ability to reason and communicate that make us extraordinary, what matter that the physical body may not be entirely whole or meet a prescribed ideal? Blindness is a physical disability. It is not a mental one.

I labored to explain all this to Aias. I labored to explain that there are as many different kinds of blindness and experiences of blindness as there are blind people in the world, that anyone can go blind but not everyone is capable of embracing the blindness and allowing it to blossom. I realized from the skeptical look on Aias's face that I was probably laboring in vain. I was failing to persuade him of things of which he had no knowledge or experience. Helen Keller understood the immensity of this task when she wrote, "It is more difficult to teach the ignorant to think than it is to teach an intelligent blind man to see the grandeur of Niagara Falls."

That evening, a particularly hot one, I went to Victor's dorm room to remind him that I wanted him to practice his English pronunciation. I had read "Stopping by Woods on a Snowy Evening" into a tape recorder for him and told him that I wanted him to memorize it and repeat it until he could recite it well enough that any English speaker in the world could recognize the words. Victor liked and understood the poem. I had realized that all three Liberians had difficulty, among their other elocutionary difficulties, in pronouncing the letter *w*. In fact, they did not pronounce it at all; they simply dropped it completely. Victor's initial attempts at the first line of the poem had sounded something like this: "Ooze oods deez ah ah fick ah noah." The ending had sounded like this: "Ah mah to go befoh ah zlip."

Victor and Johnson, his roommate, were sitting at their desks writing with their Braille slates while James, wearing nothing but shorts, lay on the floor directly beneath the cooling air current generated by the ceiling fan. James had a pillow tucked under his head and his arms crossed on his chest. Because the men were sitting in the dark, I asked their permission to turn on the light. Victor stood up and hit the light switch, and then I realized that they had all removed their big sunglasses. Johnson's eyes watered incessantly, and occasionally he wiped them with a finger. I could see a deep scar just above his right eye. James rarely removed his glasses, and he looked to me almost naked without them. He kept his eyes closed most of the time. Victor's eyes were clear, but one of them wandered freely.

"Victor," I said, "have you been practicing your pronunciation the way I asked you to do?"

He lifted a tape recorder on his desk and held it toward me. "I have been doing it."

Before I could ask him to recite the poem, James said from the floor, "He has been doing this, Auntie Rose, too many times: Ooze oods deez ah ah fick—"

I said, "*Whose.* Say it, all of you."

In unison they said, "Ooze."

"*Whose!*"

"Wooz!"

"Okay," I said. "Say *hooze.*"

"Yooz." James began to snicker nervously, but suddenly Victor hit on it. "Whose wooz deez ah ah fick—"

"*Think.*"

"Tink."

"*Th.*"

"*Ss.*"

We went on that way for quite a while, and finally I said, "Just keep listening to the recording. But really *listen* to what you're hearing and try to imitate the sounds."

Victor asked me if I had read a recent essay he had written about his life in Liberia. I had read it and told him I found it very interesting and urged him to write more. He looked surprised and pleased. "Auntie Rose, really you think I should write more?"

"I think you should all write more about yourselves," I said.

James sat up on the floor. "Even me?"

"Yes, even you. Your stories are always interesting."

Johnson said, "And what about me?"

"Of course you."

These three men had grown up in extreme poverty, and in their teens they had been subject to a terrible civil war, had been present when Liberian rebels committed unimaginably gruesome war crimes. They had had close friends and relatives murdered in front of them. Johnson's aunt had been shot. A friend of his was forced at gunpoint to rape his own aunt. He had seen small children being thrown into a deep well to drown. He had seen a pregnant woman being harassed by rebels and then, when she could not tell them whether her unborn child was a girl or a boy, heard one rebel say to another, "Let's find out." They cut the woman's belly wide open with a knife and announced "It's a girl!" as the woman lay dying. Johnson had been invited to eat boiled human flesh by some of Charles Taylor's soldiers. When he refused to eat, the soldiers said, "If you don't, we will cook you too." Despite all the terror and upheaval in their lives, the Liberian men were among the gentlest, most empathetic, and most respectful people I had ever met. They had not been hardened by their experience or filled with crippling resentment and anger. I was surprised to learn that evening that at that moment, their greatest concern was that they felt out of place at the IISE. They felt unprepared for the work that was expected of them and woefully inexperienced with computers as compared to their classmates, and they worried that their writing skills were seriously lacking because of their interrupted education. They felt, above all, that the ambitions they had had for their future work when they first arrived were ridiculously simple and modest compared to the grand ambitions of their classmates. Their classmates planned to found entire schools and social organizations; the Liberians had come here expecting to learn how to repair Braille typewriters so they could open a repair shop when they went home—they wanted to learn to do small, simple things so that they could find a way to make a living. Now they understood that typewriter repair was not something that would ever be taught at an advanced organization like this, and they were concerned that they were too far behind the others and that their ideas about their future were perhaps not entirely respected. I understood what they were telling me. They had come from nothing and now, beside the others who were generally well educated and had had better opportunities, they felt that they didn't fit in.

I explained to them, truthfully, that this idea existed only in their own heads and assured them that there was not a single person at the institute who looked down on them, that their ambitions, however small, were as worthy as anyone else's, and that their obvious intelligence and their concern for their compatriots would carry them far in their efforts to improve the lives of other blind Liberians. "Most big things start small," I said. "Many other applicants wanted the three places that you are occupying and didn't get them. The fact that you're here means that Paul and Sabriye found you worthy. It also means that you care to use your lives in the service of other people. It's not a competition. Your intention is what's important. It's all you need to get you started. Please don't be discouraged. Just take what you can from what you're being offered here and use it as best you can."

They sat, listening, as the ceiling fan chopped at the air above us. Johnson finally said, "Auntie Rose, seventy thousand people were blinded in the Liberian civil war."

Johnson affirmed this: "Seventy thousand!"

"So," I said, "there are a lot of people who need your help."

"What can we give them?" James said.

"Plenty. It doesn't matter if you don't know how to use a computer yet or spell perfectly or whether you can put a comma in the right place. The only thing that matters is what's in your heads. Just keep working and soon enough the answer will come to you," I said.

James said, "Nobody in Liberia would speak to us like that."

I asked him what he meant.

Victor said, "Nobody would encourage us."

One evening at dinner I sat at a table with Pynhoi and Hossni. At fifty-two, Hossni was the oldest student at the institute, and because of this, the others had taken to calling him Daddy. He was plump, serene, and very sweet. He was Indonesian but had lived in Saudi Arabia for years. He was a devout Muslim who prayed every day, dressed in Saudi gowns, and on special occasions wore a full Saudi headdress. Hossni's round face was almost pretty—he had fine lips and delicate features and a naturally Asian cast to his Indonesian eyes, which were deeply obscured by extremely thick eyeglasses. Like Pynhoi, Hossni could barely see. He had gradually lost most of his eyesight to a degenerative disease, and at the point that he was no longer able to continue his job because of it, he fell into a deep depression. Like many people who lose their sight as adults, Hossni found it impossible to admit to himself that he was effectively blind. He suffered a kind of paralysis of will and simply stayed at home feeling sorry for himself until one day he heard an advertisement on Saudi radio for an organization that offered training for the visually impaired. Hossni enrolled in the class, and during his seven months of training, he was astonished to discover how many blind people in his country were unemployed. Hossni was here at the IISE because he had resolved to set up his own training center for blind and visually impaired people eager to enter the profession of medical massage. Hossni's center would be the first of its kind in Saudi Arabia.

Hossni had a wife and three daughters back in Saudi Arabia. He referred to them all as "my sweethearts." That evening at dinner he told Pynhoi and me a bit about them, and Pynhoi squinted delightedly at him as he talked. His love and pride were palpable.

"Hossni," Pynhoi said, "you are a good father!"

Hossni, who was exceedingly modest, blushed and shrugged.

Pynhoi declared that her own father was also a good father and that although he did not know how to read or write, he was very intelligent. "He used to play a wooden flute and he could make music from a piece of grass." Pynhoi told us how much her parents loved animals, even though they had to kill and eat them to survive. When Pynhoi and her family were living in a village, a baby monkey got into some rice reserves and ate them. "The village people, they catch the baby monkey and tease him and torture him, and when my mother and father see this, they cry. They really cry, because all of the creatures belong to God. The people, they also used to tease me because I could not see, but my father and mother always say to them, 'You tease this girl, but she is not a stupid girl and one time she will be the one supporting the whole family!'"

Pynhoi sipped from her glass of water and then placed her arms flat on the table. She rearranged her glasses on her nose and said to Hossni, "My father was proud of me like you are proud of your girls." Pynhoi's father had died when she was seventeen. "The thing that is so sad," she said in a wondering way, "is that his life just ended."

Pynhoi told us that her mother and father would grind rice and sell it once a week in the market. Eventually Pynhoi's father had taken to sitting with the men in the market and gambling with them. He began gambling when Pynhoi was quite small, and she would sit on his shoulder and watch. "And then," Pynhoi said, "he drink some alcohol with them sometime. He would be drunk, and if my mum don't give him money for the alcohol, he scold her. But we did not have enough to eat and my mum was pregnant and we had a bad time. Sometimes my mum, she cook the rice and she don't give him any because he spend up all the money. But even though he is drunk, my father never hit my mom. Sometime she used to run and sleep in the forest to get away from him when he is drunk and scolding."

Pynhoi was such a cheerful person and seemed so happy to be alive that even as she told this story, the expression on her face and the exuberance in her strong voice had the effect of making one think, *This story is not as bad as it sounds.* It was difficult to feel terribly sad or concerned in the presence of that beaming little face, no matter what she was saying.

Pynhoi's father died when she was in the middle of her exams at a Catholic boarding school. "I was not with him, but I feel it in my body," she said. "That night I dream a fire came from the river and I say to my family, 'Get up and run from this house,' and soon as the fire from the river touch my father, he die in my dream. But really when he die they lied to me. They told me, 'Your father, he is only in the hospital.' But then when I went home they told me he is really dead."

"But what happened to him?" I said.

"He get drunk and my mom open the door and he went out. And next time later my mom she go out again and he was on the ground dead. He has vomit on his face. They all said that earlier that day he talk a lot about me and he make me a basket out of bamboo."

Pynhoi's smile had fled her face. She looked terribly worried, which was so uncharacteristic it made me feel worried. Hossni, too, looked extremely concerned. Pynhoi picked up her unused knife and fiddled with it. "I used to say to him, 'Don't drink, Father,' because when I used to come home from the boarding school he used to be always drunk, falling down this way and that way. I say to him, 'Why you so drink, Father?' He didn't help us, he was only drinking all the time and at night he opened all the doors and windows and you could see the night." Pynhoi threw her arms wide to illustrate exactly how her father opened the doors and windows, and I could almost envision the night view from the open door of their straw hut. "I say to him, 'If you drink again more I will not come home from the school to see you.' The only time I saw my father cried was when I told him I would not come home from the school again to see him."

Pynhoi stopped speaking. She held her dinner knife to within an inch of her eyeglasses to look at it. She studied it a long time, perhaps making out a small reflection of her own eye in the blade. Her face had utterly changed. Her expression was one of puzzlement and pain. She said, "My father, he cry. He say to me, 'Pynhoi, please come home to see your family. You do not have to come to see me.'"

Pynhoi put down the knife and began to cry. She slid her chair back, put one arm on the edge of the dinner table, laid her forehead on it with her face parallel to the floor, and sobbed. Hossni looked stricken. I'm certain that I did too. Hossni and I sat in shock for a full ten seconds, staring at this paragon of good cheer suddenly so over-whelmed with grief. I could see the tears dropping from Pynhoi's eyes and falling into the cupped lenses of her eyeglasses. She choked back the tears and spluttered at the floor, "I am sorry I am cry." I put my hand on her heaving back and told her that I could completely understand why she was upset, that she should not apologize for crying. Hossni also tried to comfort her. Eventually Pynhoi sat up, wiped the tears from her cheeks with the back of her hand, and confessed that she felt very guilty talking about her father this way.

"You don't have to feel guilty," I said. "If it was true, it was true. It doesn't mean your father was a bad man. Everybody has weaknesses and failings. And it doesn't mean your father didn't love you."

Pynhoi said, "Yah, Rose, I know my father love me."

"And you loved him too, right?"

She smiled. "How much!"

Pynhoi told us that her mother was now working as a laborer, hauling bricks for a mere fifty cents a day.

I had always believed that a sudden inability to see the world would be the most horrendous thing that could ever happen to me, that the magnitude of the loss would overshadow everything else in my life that had ever made me suffer. But I had begun to see that for most of the blind people I knew, there were sadnesses and tragedies far more painful than the failure of their eyes. For most of them, their blindness was not psychologically, or even practically, their greatest hardship. It did not appear to be present in their minds as the central fact about themselves. They were all frustrated and disappointed at having been marginalized, scorned, and treated with disrespect because of their blindness, and they were here because they had chosen to devote their lives to changing that and similar discriminations, to battling ignorance and the hatreds that arise from it. But they were human beings just like the rest of us, with lives and important relationships and personal complications that from time to time took precedence over everything else. Just like the rest of us.

As I was getting up from the table to get some more rice, I saw Jayne approaching the stage at the end of the dining room. She leaned over a bit and considered the step up carefully before she took it, and then she turned to face the room. "Everyone!" she shouted. "Listen to me! I have an announcement to make. One of our colleagues is celebrating a birthday. Can you all help to sing the happy-birthday song?"

The room went silent. As she spoke, Jayne held her hands clasped before her at arm's length, fingers intertwined, in a posture of pleading. She announced that she would not reveal who the birthday person was but that when we reached the point in the song at which the name was usually mentioned, we should just fill the space in by singing "Hmmm-hmmm-hmmm." "And," Jayne said, "when we reach 'how-old-are-you-now,' we will let the birthday person stand up and tell us how old she is!"

Jayne began to sing the song, and the rest of us, somewhat puzzled, joined in. After a few phrases, Jayne planted her hands on her hips and shouted in impatience and displeasure, "Wait a minute! Stop! Will you all *please* try to sing it musically?"

Jayne's confident bossiness was so charming and her intent so heartfelt that it was impossible for anyone to protest. We started the song over, and when we reached the point at which the celebrant is addressed by name, we did as we were instructed and somewhat ridiculously hummed the notes of the song. As we sang, someone flipped off the dining room lights, and the kitchen staff came out carrying a large birthday cake lit with a single candle and placed it on the serving table. At the song's end, we waited for the birthday person to stand up. Finally Pynhoi got slowly out of her chair and went to the table with her hands pressed over her mouth. She leaned over, her face aglow in the candlelight, and examined the cake, scanning it carefully through her glasses, and when she realized that it had the words *Happy Birthday, Pynhoi* written on it in pink icing, she gasped in disbelief and delight and hugged herself. Someone handed her a large knife and instructed her to cut the cake. Instead, Pynhoi began to pace back and forth in front of the table, waving the knife as she talked.

"Oh. I do not know what to say. Oh, thank you very much. I am twenty-four years old today. Yes, I am twenty-four years old now. And, you know, I do not know what to say. I don't know. Because I have never before celebrated my birthday. Because my mother did not have the money to celebrate for all four of her children or to buy a cake. So, this is the first time ever in my life anyone celebrates my birthday. This is my first birthday cake."

Pynhoi was beside herself. And again she began to cry. She raised the hand that held the big cake knife to the side of her mouth, and she kept it there awkwardly as she continued to talk. "I am so happy here. Oh. You have been very generous to me. This morning I did not know it was the seventeenth. Jayne, she come to me and said, 'Pynhoi, it is something special day today.' I had to look at the calendar to see that it is really my birthday." With her free hand, Pynhoi wiped her tears, which were now furiously falling. "And so, everybody, my friends, I will call my mother on the telephone and tell her that you have really given me a cake and your love and goodwill will go all over the world and spread to other people."

Pynhoi was so overcome, she bent over to hide her face for a moment. Then she straightened, said, "I am so lucky," and turned toward the cake to begin cutting it. I got up and explained to her that it was a tradition that she make a wish and then blow out the candle on the cake. She seemed not to understand it. "Wish for something, Pynhoi. Then lean over and blow the candle out with your breath and the wish will come true."

She laughed, thought, then blew with all her might. The candle went out, and for a couple of seconds, we found ourselves bathed in beautiful darkness.

# Author's Note

In researching this book, I spent a great deal of time with many students at Braille Without Borders, in Lhasa, in 2005, and at the International Institute for Social Entrepreneurs, in Trivandrum, Kerala, in 2009. This book is based on my extensive notes on my experiences and, in some cases, on recorded classes and formal interviews. To protect individuals' privacy, I have changed some of the names here.

# Acknowledgments

I am grateful to Sabriye Tenberken and Paul Kronenberg for welcoming me so warmly at Braille Without Borders in Lhasa and at the International Institute for Social Entrepreneurs, now known as Kanthari, in Kerala. Over the past eight years I have learned a great deal from these two gifted, spirited people. I am also fortunate to have worked with their colleagues Nora Hartenstein, Isabel Torres Cruzado, Arky Rekesh Ambati, and Amjad Prawej. I am further indebted to all the blind and partially sighted children and adults I worked with in Lhasa and Kerala. Their good humor, empathy, resilience, and dynamism make them superb teachers.

I would like to thank John Barnett, the brilliant book designer, for his innovative ideas; Madeleine Stein for her early reading; Tracy Roe for her excellent copyediting; Barbara Kennedy Roney for her generosity and her serene and forbearing ear; Kate Wodehouse at the Providence Athenaeum for helping me find the von Senden book; Pat Towers for sending me to Tibet for *O, The Oprah Magazine;* the John Simon Guggenheim Foundation for their financial support; and Aias Dimaratos Tchacos for his *paramythia* and other Greek diversions.

I cannot acknowledge enough my literary agent, Betsy Lerner, for her twenty-seven years of friendship, sound literary advice, and moral support; or my editor, Pat Strachan, for her faithful encouragement, her keen editorial logic, and her patience with what must for a couple of years have seemed a project without end.

# Bibliography

The following is a list of some of the books and essays that I found useful in my research for this project. Three books that were of invaluable help and interest to me were Zina Weygand's history *The Blind in French Society from the Middle Ages to the Century of Louis Braille,* Elisabeth Gitter's biography *The Imprisoned Guest: Samuel Howe and Laura Bridgman, the Original Deaf-Blind Girl,* and Robert Kurson's *Crashing Through: A True Story of Risk, Adventure, and the Man Who Dared to See.* I owe these three authors an especial debt of gratitude.

Barasch, Moshe. *Blindness: The History of a Mental Image in Western Thought.* New York: Routledge, 2001.

Clark, Eleanor. *Eyes, Etc.: A Memoir.* New York: Pantheon, 1977.

Derrida, Jacques. *Memoirs of the Blind: The Self-Portrait and Other Ruins.* Translated by Pascale-Anne Brault and Michael Naas. Chicago: University of Chicago Press, 1993.

Dickens, Charles. *American Notes for General Circulation.* CreateSpace Independent Publishing Platform, 2011.

Diderot, Denis. *Early Philosophical Works.* Edited and translated by Margaret Jourdain. London: Open Court, 1916.

Freeburg, Ernest. *The Education of Laura Bridgman: First Deaf and Blind Person to Learn Language.* Cambridge, MA: Harvard University Press, 2001.

French, Richard S. *From Homer to Helen Keller.* New York: American Foundation for the Blind, 1932.

Gitter, Elisabeth. *The Imprisoned Guest: Samuel Howe and Laura Bridgman, the Original Deaf-Blind Girl.* New York: Farrar, Straus and Giroux, 2001.

Gregory, R. L. *Eye and Brain: The Psychology of Seeing.* Fifth Edition. Princeton, NJ: Princeton University Press, 1990.

_____. "Recovery from Early Blindness: A Case Study," in *Concepts and Mechanisms of Perception.* New York: Charles Scribner's Sons, 1974.

Haüy, Valentin. *An Essay on the Education of the Blind.* Edinburgh: Alexander Chapman, 1793.

Herrmann, Dorothy. *Helen Keller: A Life.* New York: Alfred A. Knopf, 1998.

Howe, Samuel Gridley. *Annual Reports of the Trustees of the Perkins Institution and Massachusetts Asylum for the Blind.* Disability History Museum Online Library. http://www.disabilitymuseum.org/dhm/lib/detail.html?id=2295.

_____. *Education of the Blind.* London: Samson Lowe, Marston. Digitizing sponsor: National Federation of the Blind.

Hull, John M. *Touching the Rock: An Experience of Blindness.* New York: Vintage Books, 1990.

Keller, Helen. *The Story of My Life.* Edited by Roger Shattuck with Dorothy Herrmann. New York: W. W. Norton, 2003.

_____. *The World I Live In and Optimism: A Collection of Essays.* Mineola, NY: Dover Publications, 2009.

Kleege, Georgina. *Blind Rage: Letters to Helen Keller.* Washington, DC: Gallaudet University Press, 2006.

_____. *Sight Unseen.* New Haven, CT: Yale University Press, 1999.

Kurson, Robert. *Crashing Through: A True Story of Risk, Adventure, and the Man Who Dared to See.* New York: Random House, 2007.

Kuusisto, Stephen. *Planet of the Blind: A Memoir.* New York: Delta, 1999.

Lusseyran, Jacques. *And There Was Light: Autobiography of Jacques Lusseyran, Blind Hero of the French Resistance.* Translated by Elizabeth R. Cameron. New York: Parabola Books, 1998.

Mehta, Ved. *Vedi.* New York: Oxford University Press, 1981.

Meltzer, Milton. *A Light in the Dark: The Life of Samuel Gridley Howe.* Cleveland: Modern Curriculum Press, 1964.

Sacks, Oliver. *An Anthropologist on Mars: Seven Paradoxical Tales.* New York: Alfred A. Knopf, 1995.

———. *The Mind's Eye.* New York: Alfred A. Knopf, 2010.

Sanford, E. C. *The Writings of Laura Bridgman.* San Francisco: Overland Monthly, 1887.

Scott, Robert A. *The Making of Blind Men.* New York: Russell Sage Foundation, 1969.

Tenberken, Sabriye. *My Path Leads to Tibet: The Inspiring Story of How One Young Blind Woman Brought Hope to the Blind Children of Tibet.* New York: Arcade Publishing, 2003.

von Senden, Marius. *Space and Sight: The Perception of Space and Shape in the Congenitally Blind Before and After Operation.* Translated by Peter Heath. London: Methuen, 1960.

Weygand, Zina. *The Blind in French Society from the Middle Ages to the Century of Louis Braille.* Translated by Emily-Jane Cohen. Stanford: Stanford University Press, 2009.

# Index

# About the Author

Rosemary Mahoney is the author of *Down the Nile: Alone in a Fisherman's Skiff,* a *New York Times* Notable Book; *Whoredom in Kimmage: The World of Irish Women,* a National Book Critics Circle Award finalist; *A Likely Story: One Summer with Lillian Hellman; The Early Arrival of Dreams: A Year in China,* a *New York Times* Notable Book; and *The Singular Pilgrim: Travels on Sacred Ground.* She is the recipient of a Whiting Writers' Award, a grant from the National Endowment for the Arts, and a 2011 Guggenheim Fellowship. She is a citizen of the Republic of Ireland and the United States. She lives in Rhode Island.